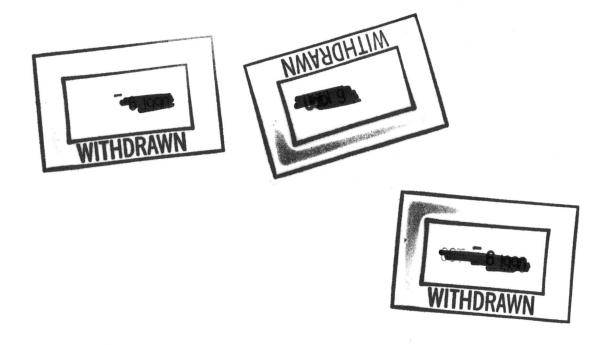

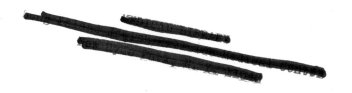

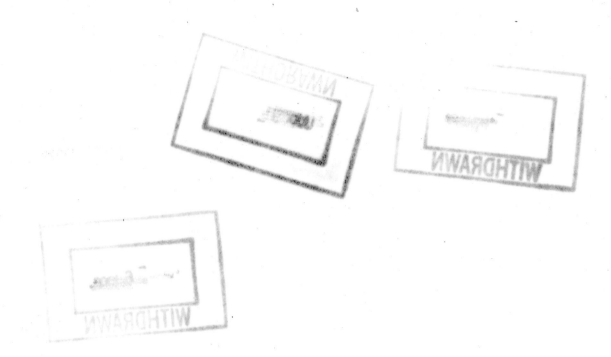

# Atlas of the Ocular Fundus

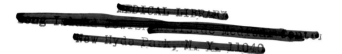

# Atlas of the Ocular Fundus

Photographs of Typical Changes in Ocular and
Systemic Disease

Hans Sautter, MD, Professor,
Director of the University Eye-Clinic Hamburg

Wolfgang Straub, MD, Professor,
Director of the University Eye-Clinic Marburg

Hermann Roßmann, MD,
University Eye-Clinic Hamburg

Second, revised Edition
327 Illustrations, mostly in color

#4957

J. B. Lippincott Comp. · Philadelphia 1977

*Authors' addresses:*

Professor Dr. med. Dr. h. c. *Hans Sautter,* Director of the University Eye-Clinic, Martini-straße 52, D-2000 Hamburg 20.

Professor Dr. med. Dr. h. c. *Wolfgang Straub,* Director of the University Eye-Clinic, Robert-Koch-Straße 4, D-3550 Marburg.

Dr. med. *Hermann Roßmann,* Wissenschaftlicher Oberrat, University Eye-Clinic, Martini-straße 52, D-2000 Hamburg 20.

*Translated into English by*

Dr. med. E. N. Hinzpeter, Tangstedter Landstraße 400, D-2000 Hamburg 62.


Distributed in North America by J. B. Lippincott Company, Philadelphia, Pennsylvania 19105.


The 1st edition was published in 1963 in German. Title: Sautter/Straub, Der photographierte Augenhintergrund. ISBN 3-541-02461-5.


ISBN 0-397-58213-7                                                                            76-488 79


© Urban & Schwarzenberg, München–Wien–Baltimore 1977 (ISBN 3-541-02462-3)

Printed in Germany by Kastner & Callwey, Buch- und Offsetdruckerei, München.

# Preface

The following collection represents a wider aspect of the previous publication "The photographed fundus of the eye" by *Sautter* and *Straub* written in German in 1963.

Ophthalmology is a visual discipline. In order to recognize and interpret pathological changes correctly, it is important for the clinician to compare his own observations with a typical picture of the disease in question. We have endeavoured to present not only lesions which have priority interest for the ophthalmologist, but also conditions with diagnostic significance for general systemic diseases especially of the vascular system which the internist and general practitioner are likely to meet in their daily practice. Funduscopy also plays an important part in the diagnosis and treatment of neurological and neurosurgical diseases, and we believe that this atlas will also be useful to specialists in these fields. Last but not least, we hope that this book will interest and aid scientific workers.

It was impossible to divide the various subjects into a rigid system. But we have tried to place related diseases in close sequence. Aspects of treatment have also been considered in so far as they appeared necessary in this context.

We wish to thank the photographers of the University Eye-Clinic in Hamburg and Marburg, Fräulein Hadlock and Frau Ursprung respectively. We should also like to thank Dr. Hinzpeter for translating the text into English.

We are especially grateful to Mr. Michael Urban and Dr. Degkwitz of the publishers Urban & Schwarzenberg for their kind help and advice in publishing this book.

*Hans Sautter*
*Wolfgang Straub*
*Hermann Roßmann*

V

# Contents

# The fundus of experimental animals used in ophthalmology

# The fundus of experimental animals

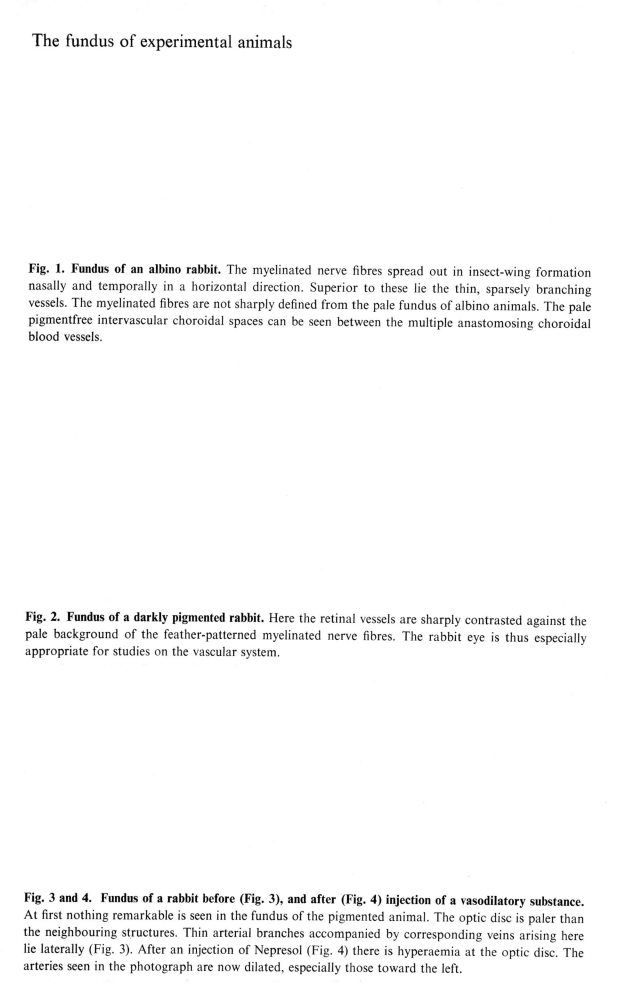

**Fig. 1. Fundus of an albino rabbit.** The myelinated nerve fibres spread out in insect-wing formation nasally and temporally in a horizontal direction. Superior to these lie the thin, sparsely branching vessels. The myelinated fibres are not sharply defined from the pale fundus of albino animals. The pale pigmentfree intervascular choroidal spaces can be seen between the multiple anastomosing choroidal blood vessels.

**Fig. 2. Fundus of a darkly pigmented rabbit.** Here the retinal vessels are sharply contrasted against the pale background of the feather-patterned myelinated nerve fibres. The rabbit eye is thus especially appropriate for studies on the vascular system.

**Fig. 3 and 4. Fundus of a rabbit before (Fig. 3), and after (Fig. 4) injection of a vasodilatory substance.** At first nothing remarkable is seen in the fundus of the pigmented animal. The optic disc is paler than the neighbouring structures. Thin arterial branches accompanied by corresponding veins arising here lie laterally (Fig. 3). After an injection of Nepresol (Fig. 4) there is hyperaemia at the optic disc. The arteries seen in the photograph are now dilated, especially those toward the left.

2

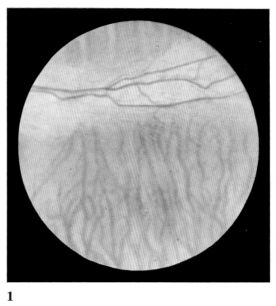

1

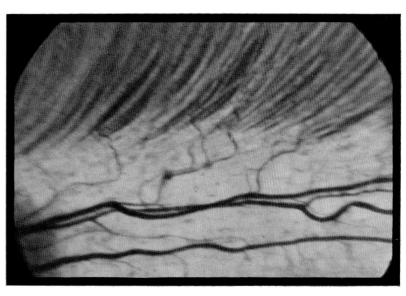

2

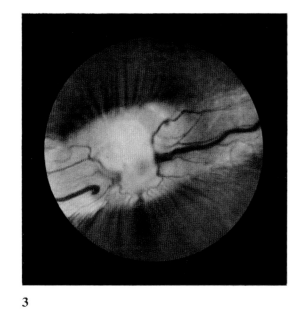

3

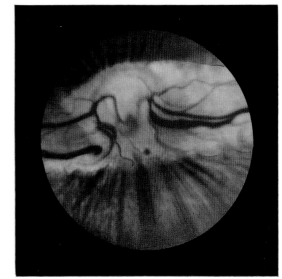

4

3

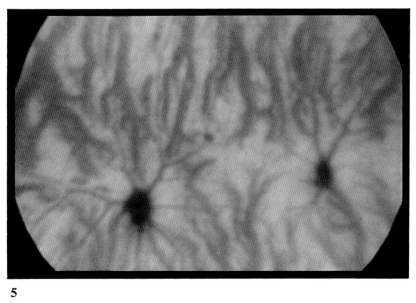

**5**

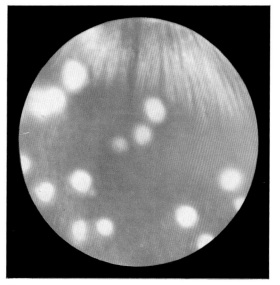

**6**

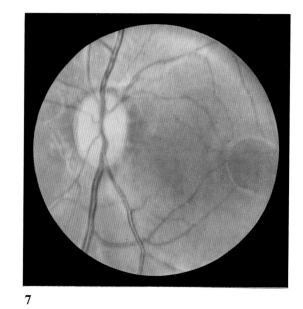

**7**

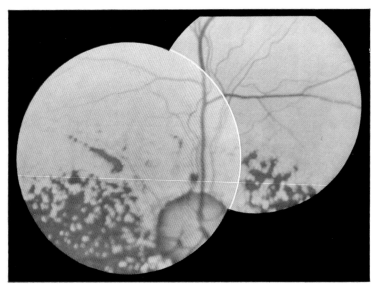

**8**

4

**Fig. 5. Fundus of a rabbit after an experiment with vital dye.** Vascular studies of the fundus can also be carried out with vital dyes. Shown is isolated filling of choroidal vessels in an albino animal after injection of Trypan Blue. The vessels are coloured brown. The exits of the vortex veins show up as dark points.

**Fig. 6. Experimentally induced, Candida albicans mycotic fundus changes in a rabbit.** An injection was given 4 days ago, of Candida albicans in the auricular vein (1,3 mg/kg body weight). 3 days later several round, lightly coloured foci, which increase in intensity up to the 5th day, appeared.

**Fig. 7. Fundus of a 6-month-old rhesus monkey.** The optic nerve disc and the vascular pattern correspond almost completely to that of the human. Note the peculiar olive-green reflecting young fundus with contrasting fovea centralis.

**Fig. 8. Fundus of an adult dog (Pomeranian).** The extremely bright reflecting, and in some areas coloured, surfaces around and above the optic nerve disc represent the tapetum lucidum. It is demarcated from the rest of the fundus by an intensely pigmented border. The almost violet colour of the optic nerve disc is remarkable as in some places is the practically perpendicular branching of the retinal vessels.

# The normal fundus of the human eye

**Fig. 9. Normal fundus; left eye.** The reddish colouring of the normal fundus (i.e. free from pathological change) is dependent on the circulation, especially the blood content of the choriocapillary system; the pigment content of the choroid (and thus the racial characteristics of the individual); the nature of the pigment epithelium; the form of the light source used for examination; and (especially for subtle differences in the periphery) the age of the individual.

Here one sees the regular red colouring of an averagely pigmented European. The physiological excavation of the optic disc is visible. The rest of the optic disc lies in the same plane as the retina. The vessels are normal as regards their exit, their pattern and their ramifications. The veins and arteries divide into their main branches at the optic disc. The fact that the retinal vessels do not anastomose with one another is of great functional significance.

**Fig. 10. Normal fundus of a 30-year-old Indonesian; right eye.** Fundus of a rather darkly pigmented individual. The nerve fibre layer is distinctly visible especially in the region of the upper and lower vascular arc. The central fundus stands out in sharp colour contrast from its surroundings. The area known as the central area or macula lutea is a horizontally oval region more intensely coloured than its surroundings, with a central pit known as the fovea centralis.

The macula lutea is named after the yellow colouring in this area in the eye of a corpse and is not seen when the fundus is visualized with normal light. The axial reflexes seen here and there along the arteries and veins, result from the light reflex of the cylindrical blood column. These reflexes are only seen along the retinal vessels and therefore aid in the differentiation to choroidal vessels. The band reflexes on either side of the veins and arteries seen in children and in young persons but not later, result from the concave cylindrical grooves on either side of the vessels, which are slightly raised above the level of the retina.

**Fig. 11. Normal fundus visualized with a light source of 507 mμ wavelength.** The visualisation in redfree light is important for the examination of the central fundus. Vogt pointed out that the choroid becomes practically invisible in redfree light because the retina reflects so much light that relatively little can penetrate to the uvea. Due to the light filter in the following case, the arteries and veins stand out in sharp contrast: the arteries appear grey, the veins almost black. The multiple reflexes of the youthful fundus (16 year old) are easily recognizable.

**Fig. 12. Normal fundus visualized with light of 580 mμ wavelength.** Light of this particular wavelength appears especially suitable for demonstrating the smaller vessels. One can see small branching vessels especially temporal to the optic disc running towards the macula. Here the arteries appear violet and the veins are slightly darker. The posterior pole of this 15 year old visualized in yellow, redfree light is sharply demarcated and reflects a greenish tone.

**Fig. 13. Tabulated fundus of a 54-year-old woman (strongly pigmented brunette); right eye.** The reflexes decrease with increasing age. The pigment contrast between the intervascular spaces and the blood vessels is greater. The walls of the retinal vessels show no reflexes, and the fundus on the whole develops a dull appearance. Added to this in the picture are a small temporal conus and a slightly slanting optic disc corresponding to a minimal myopia.

**Fig. 14. Fundus flavus; right eye.** Compared with the types described above, the intervascular spaces of the choroid have a lighter colouring here than the choroidal vessels themselves. Due to paucity of pigment, retinal vessels have no contrasting background so that their colouring is similar to that of the choroid. The functionally important central area of the fundus possesses a better distribution of choroidal vessels than the neighbouring areas. Normally 2 reflexes are present at the posterior pole: the more or less distinct ridgelike macula reflex (wallreflex), and the dot or crescent-shaped, usually very bright foveolar reflex. In this picture the wall reflex has a double contour corresponding to the width of the ridge present.

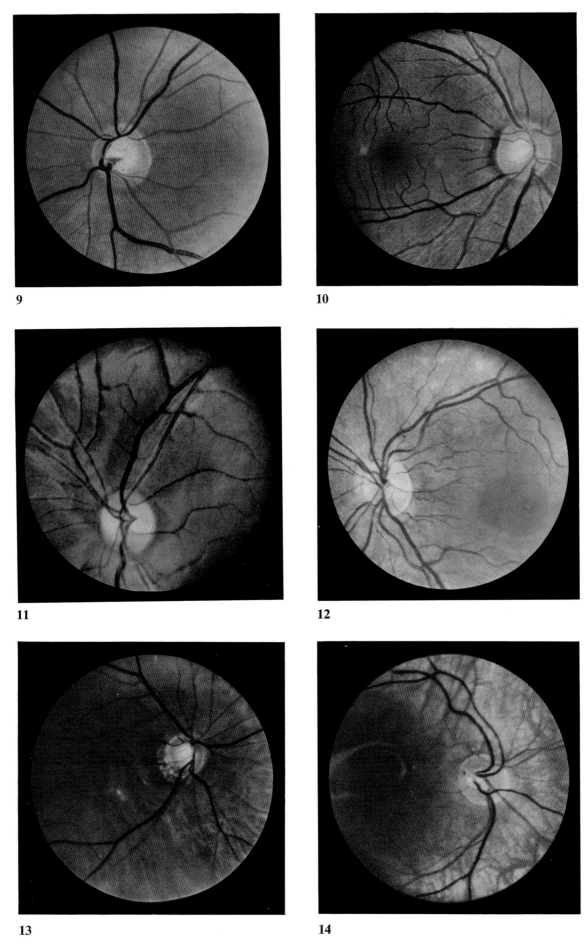

9

10

11

12

13

14

# Physiological variants and congenital malformations

**Fig. 15. Dysversion of the disc with cilio-retinal artery; right eye.** Distinctly tabulated fundus of a 22 year old. The optic disc appears slanting and oval in form instead of its usual almost round contour. A further, not infrequent anomaly, is the cilio-retinal artery. In this case it commences at the temporal lower border of the optic disc and follows a downward course. These vessels can play an important role functionally under certain pathological conditions, as they are not branches of the central retinal artery. Whereas the central artery arises directly from the ophthalmic artery and enters the optic nerve approximately 10–15 mm behind the lamina cribrosa, the cilio-retinal arteries arise from the circle of Zinn which is fed by the posterior ciliary arteries. They do not run within the optic nerve but within its sheaths.

**Fig. 16. Dysversion of the optic disc; right eye.** This anomaly of the optic disc is frequently found in association with myopia, astigmatism and (or) congenitally poor vision. This 12-year-old patient has normal visual acuity. The upper half of the oval slanting optic disc appears to partly cover the lower portion. The main vessels arise centrally, curving over the ridge superiorly; whereas the inferior arteries and veins follow a stretched course. Tabulated fundus.

**Fig. 17 and 18. Pseudo-papilloedema with hypermetropia; right and left eye of the same patient.** Due to the short axis of the eye in hypermetropia, partial or complete blurring of the disc margins can occur. In this 16-year-old patient blurred margins of the disc are present bilaterally and over the whole circumference. Important in the differential diagnosis to true papilloedema are the lack of venous congestion and haemorrhages and the fact that the fundus picture remained unchanged over repeated examinations. Vision in both eyes was 5/5 with a correction of +4,0.
Occasionally a pseudo-papilloedema is seen with myopia. The increased growth of the eyeball occurs mainly in an axial direction. At first there is a thinning out of the fundus between the macula and the disc with compression nasal to this. According to the influence of the stretching or compressing forces, a blurring of the whole disc can occur. If the compression only occurs nasal to the optic disc during the growth in axial length of the globe, then the blurring of the disc margin will only occur in this area.

**Fig. 19 and 20. Drusen of the optic disc; right and left eye of the same patient.** Hyaline masses in the region of the disc sometimes appear as glittering formations. One can recognize them here on both sides at the inferior nasal margin of the optic disc. There is often a blurring of the disc margins as well as a certain amount of prominence. The drusen disc is important in the differential diagnoses of a true papilloedema or an optic neuritis. Thorough examinations allow an ophthalmological differentiation. Recently there is a belief that the drusen disc is of pathological significance as a deposition of colloidal substances. Such cases one can regard not as congenital abnormalities but rather as secondary changes.

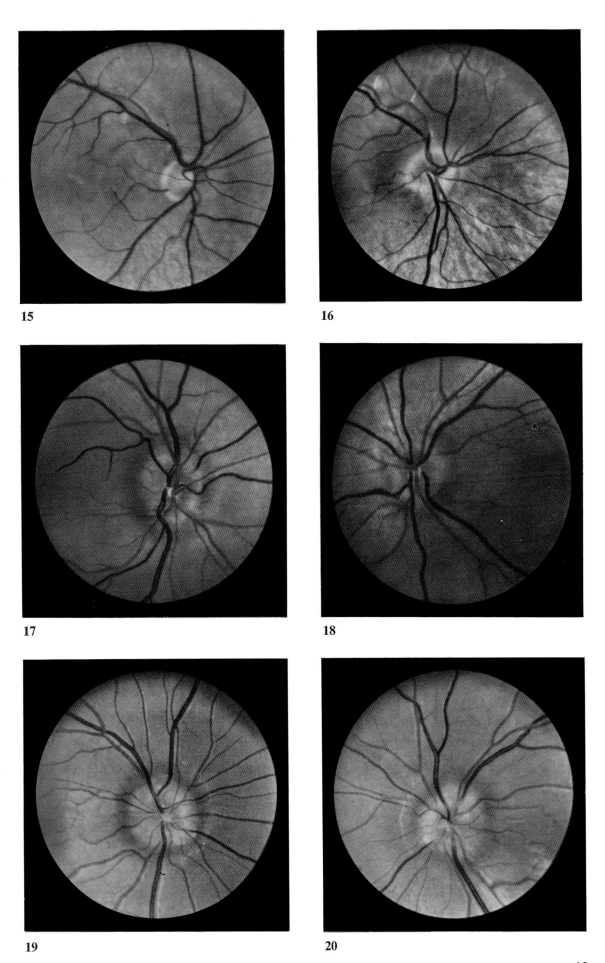

15

16

17

18

19

20

13

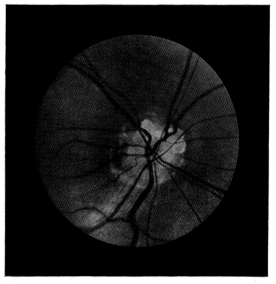

**21**

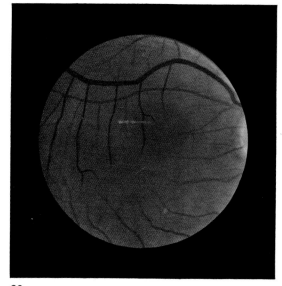

**22**

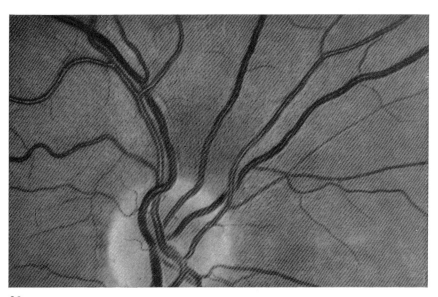

**23**

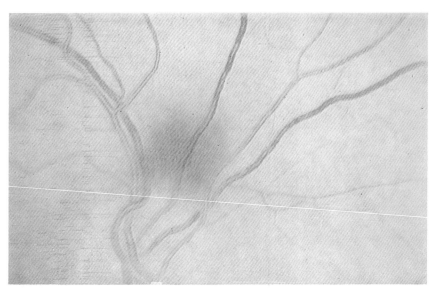

**24**

**Fig. 21. Drusen of the optic disc; right eye.** Here one can see the drusen at the upper and upper nasal optic margin as round glittering structures giving the optic disc a mulberry appearance. The rest of the circumference has no drusen. The eye of this 48-year-old patient was functionally normal.

**Fig. 22. Naevus of the choroid of a 60-year-old patient; right eye.** Directly nasally and above the macula is a choroidal naevus the size of an optic disc, with uninvolved branches of retinal vessels coursing over it. Naevi as in this case are usually discovered by chance. However, they still necessitate exact and repeated examination because some of them can develop malignant properties. A point in favour of a benign naevus and against malignant change is the absence of prominence of the overlying retina seen on repeated examination with the triple-mirror, Goldmann contact glass and the Gullstrand ophthalmoscope. In the picture here, one can see the vascular supply to the posterior pole. There is a remarkably stretched almost palisade pattern of the arterial and venous branches arising superiorly as an expression of the onset of arteriosclerotic circulatory disorders. Added to this is the absent macular reflex and the increased (senile) tabulation of the choroid.

**Fig. 23. Naevus of the choroid; right eye.** Immediately above the optic disc is a choroidal naevus (benign melanoma) approximately the size of an optic disc, over which the course of the retinal vessels remains unchanged. This naevus also remained stationary over several years.

**Fig. 24. Infrared photography of the choroidal naevus shown in Fig. 23.** This method of photography which depends on longwave infrared light helps to establish the diagnosis: a subretinal haemorrhage would show a brownish colouring here instead of the black pigmentation of a naevus.

**Fig. 25. Choroidal naevus; left eye.** In this case it is much more difficult to believe that the naevus is benign although the condition has remained unchanged over several years. The naevus encompasses the lower portion of the optic disc which has thus lost its circular form. It consists of two differently pigmented zones: a very dark black central area and a less pigmented almost triangular peripheral region. The position as well as the appearance of the central zone arouses the suspicion of malignancy. This 53-year-old female patient is under constant observation.

**Fig. 26. Choroidal naevus; right eye.** This pigmented naevus situated in the region of the temporal superior retinal vein has remained stationary since 1957. Hypertensive vascular changes are also visible in the fundus of this 64-year-old female patient: i.e. irregularly calibrated, segmentally narrowed arteries with increased reflexes, and tortuosity of the veins and venules. The nasal and superior margins of the optic nerve disc are blurred (pseudopapilloedema). Visual acuity $+1,0 = 5/4$.

**Fig. 27. Naevoid retinal pigmentation; left eye.** Note the increased circumscribed pigmentary deposits in the retina. Generally speaking these foci are multiple, strongly pigmented, sharply demarcated and of a small size. As in this case they usually are a chance finding and do not require further examination.

**Fig. 28. Myelinated nerve fibres; left eye.** The myelinated nerve fibres represent a stationary congenital anomaly, whereby the optic nerve fibres fail to shed their myelin sheaths at their exit from the lamina cribrosa. The result is flame-shaped white spots with feathery endings. The retinal vessels are mostly invisible here, though in some places their course runs superior to the myelinated fibres. In this patient the optic disc is surrounded on all sides except at its temporal inferior margin by myelinated nerve fibres of varying length.

**Fig. 29. Myelinated nerve fibres in the right eye of a Chinese.** Apart from the myelinated nerve fibres around the exit of the main vascular branches at the superior and inferior optic disc margins (less marked than in the previous case), one can see the racially characteristic yellow-brownish colour of the fundus. The intervascular pigmented spaces of the choroid are clearly visible, as is a small cilio-retinal artery at the temporal margin of the optic disc.

**Fig. 30. Myelinated nerve fibres; right eye.** The cometlike dense myelinated sheaths which spread out in all directions corresponding to the retinal nerve fibre pattern, can resemble an ischaemic retinal oedema with retinal arterial branch occlusion. However, contrary to the latter, myelinated nerve fibres usually cover the vessels completely.

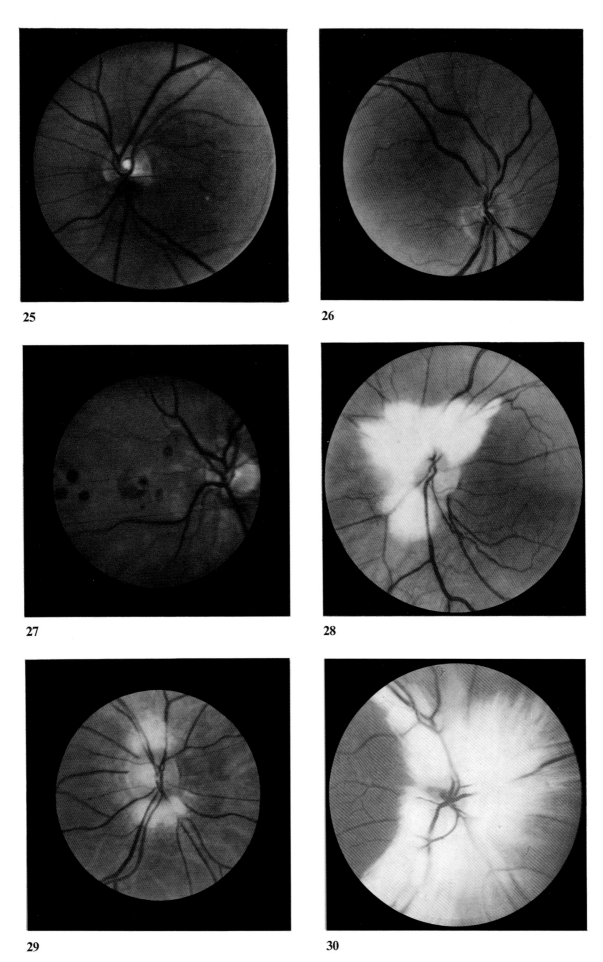

25

26

27

28

29

30

17

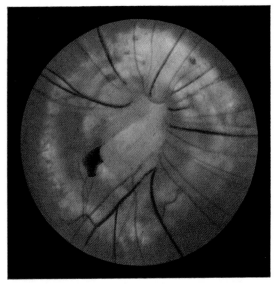

**31**

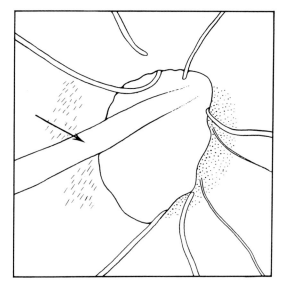

**31a**

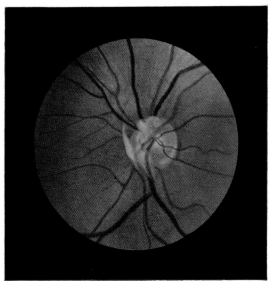

**32**

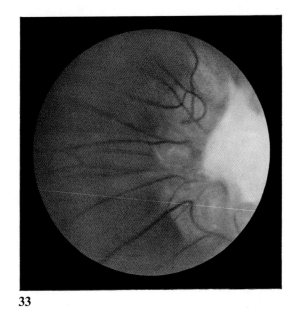

**33**

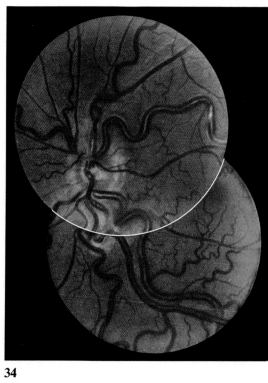

**34**

18

**Fig. 31. Coloboma of the optic disc with remnants of the vitreal artery; right eye.** Extreme malformation of the optic disc, caused by failure in fusion of the foetal cleft of the optic vesicle between the fifth and sixth week of embryonic life. The optic disc can be replaced by glial mesodermal tissue in such cases. The vessels bend out over the central conelike excavation along the whole circumference of the optic disc. Surrounding the central excavation is a zone in which the choroid is absent, and where the pale sclera is visible interrupted by a slight irregular pigmentation. This region is framed by a ring of bone-corpuscular-like pigment spots that are reminiscent of a tapetoretinal degeneration. Temporal and inferior to the optic disc there are fibrous remnants of the hyaloid artery (sketch), which is another indication of embryonic maldevelopment. Frequently in such cases there are further, more deeply situated malformations of the embryonic eye anlage, so that the vessels seen here are probably mostly retino-ciliary veins and cilio-retinal arteries respectively. The malformation results in a diminished visual acuity of 3/100.

**Fig. 32. Delicate epipapillary membrane; left eye.** On the nasal half of the optic disc, and running onto the retina, lies a fine pale tissue which veils the inferior vessels at the disc margin.

**Fig. 33. Epipapillary membrane; right eye.** In contrast to the previous case, here the whole optic disc is veiled. The membrane consists of varying dense zones, a central button-like, prominent, snow-white nucleus surrounded by a grey border which follows the vascular pattern in some places. In this area the atypically distributed, mostly cilio-retinal or retino-ciliary vessels originate. Here is a case of embryonal tissue remnants which occur in connection with a disturbed involution of the hyaloid artery. The malformation in this patient was accompanied by a diminished visual acuity to mere perception of light.

**Fig. 34. Tortuositas vasorum; left eye.** Note dilatation and increased varicosity of the veins and arteries. The temporal superior and inferior vessels are especially involved and show broad axial reflecting lines. The absence of signs of stasis, the unaltered picture over repeated examination, and the normal condition of the patient characterizes this as a congenital anomaly. Visual acuity is normal, and there are no other functional defects.

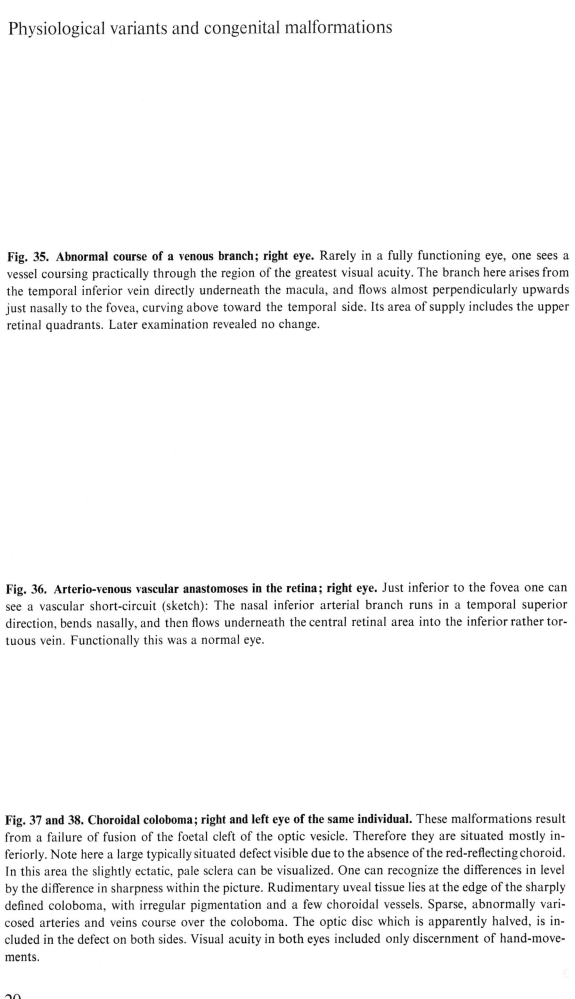

**Fig. 35. Abnormal course of a venous branch; right eye.** Rarely in a fully functioning eye, one sees a vessel coursing practically through the region of the greatest visual acuity. The branch here arises from the temporal inferior vein directly underneath the macula, and flows almost perpendicularly upwards just nasally to the fovea, curving above toward the temporal side. Its area of supply includes the upper retinal quadrants. Later examination revealed no change.

**Fig. 36. Arterio-venous vascular anastomoses in the retina; right eye.** Just inferior to the fovea one can see a vascular short-circuit (sketch): The nasal inferior arterial branch runs in a temporal superior direction, bends nasally, and then flows underneath the central retinal area into the inferior rather tortuous vein. Functionally this was a normal eye.

**Fig. 37 and 38. Choroidal coloboma; right and left eye of the same individual.** These malformations result from a failure of fusion of the foetal cleft of the optic vesicle. Therefore they are situated mostly inferiorly. Note here a large typically situated defect visible due to the absence of the red-reflecting choroid. In this area the slightly ectatic, pale sclera can be visualized. One can recognize the differences in level by the difference in sharpness within the picture. Rudimentary uveal tissue lies at the edge of the sharply defined coloboma, with irregular pigmentation and a few choroidal vessels. Sparse, abnormally varicosed arteries and veins course over the coloboma. The optic disc which is apparently halved, is included in the defect on both sides. Visual acuity in both eyes included only discernment of hand-movements.

20

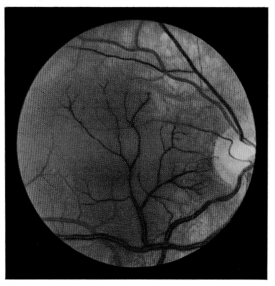

35

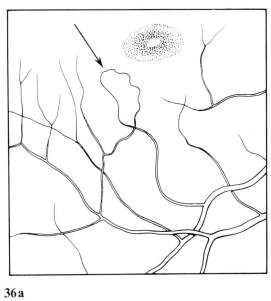

36 a

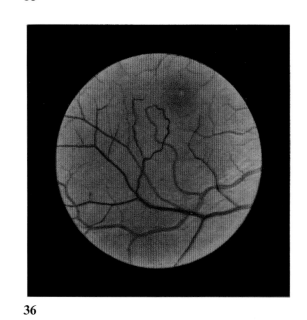

36

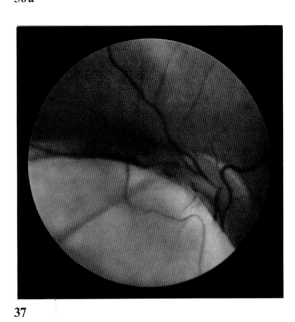

37

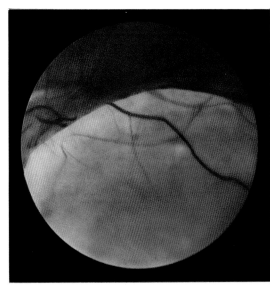

38

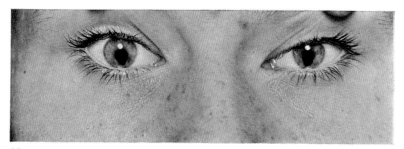

**39**

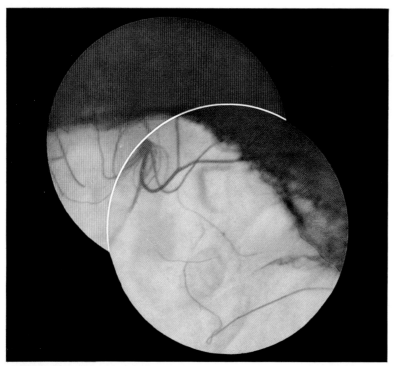

**40**

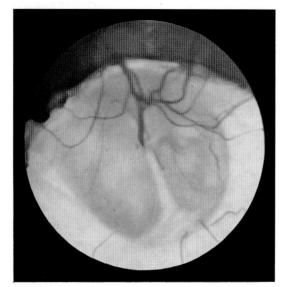

**41**

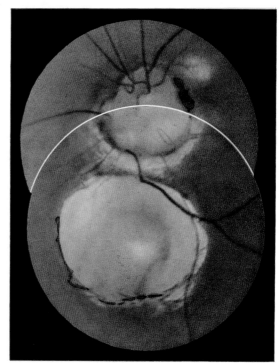

**42**

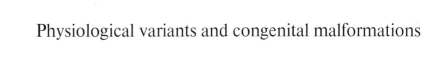

**Fig. 39–41. Iris and choroid coloboma; right and left eye of the same individual.** Coloboma can involve the iris alone, or can stretch from the posterior choroid to the iris anteriorly. The defect is typically in the inferior nasal quadrant (Fig. 39). The optic disc in both eyes (Fig. 40 and 41) is situated at the superior edge of the coloboma. The edges are hardly visible. Occasional atypical retinal vessels stretch across the pale area of the coloboma and show up the difference in level of the coloboma and the surrounding retina. On the left (Fig. 41) the macula is included in the defect. Visual acuity in this 14-year-old patient was on the right 5/25, on the left counting of fingers in 1 m. Histological studies have shown that the retina is present as a rudimentary glial layer in the area of the coloboma.

**Fig. 42. Rudimentary choroidal coloboma and coloboma of the optic nerve; left eye.** Instead of the optic disc there is an irregularly formed excavation into whose upper margin a few sparse vessels enter. At the lower edge are a few cilio-retinal arteries and cilio-retinal veins respectively. Beneath the optic nerve coloboma bounded by a halo-like border, lies a narrow bridge of normal choroidal tissue. The rudimentary circular choroidal coloboma does not extend to the periphery. Visual acuity of this eye is 1/35.

**Fig. 43. So-called macula coloboma; right eye.** Atypical coloboma of the choroid probably result from an atypical position of the foetal cleft. Here one finds not infrequently the so-called macula coloboma. A bridge of normal tissue lies between the optic nerve disc and the defect which does not extend to the periphery. In this case the large defect which was discovered in childhood has a strongly pigmented lower border and a superior ridge, which is practically bounded by the temporal superior vascular arc. Recent investigations have shown that the clinical picture of so-called macula coloboma can be caused by an intrauterine inflammation e.g. toxoplasmosis; so that not all cases are the result of true congenital malformations. The formation of a macula coloboma in an otherwise normal eye is difficult to explain embryologically. In our patient too the clinical features are against a true malformation. A toxoplasmotic infection could not be verified.

**Fig. 44. Large physiological cupping of the optic nerve disc; left eye.** Frequently as a variation to the norm, the nerve fibres diverge before entering the lamina cribrosa, and this results in a pale central, but not marginal, deep cup on the optic nerve disc: the physiological cup. In this case the vessels are located nasally. One can discern the sieve-like lamina cribrosa in the depths of the cup.

**Fig. 45 and 46. Cupping of the optic disc in myopia, with absence of raised intraocular pressure; right and left eye of the same 71-year-old patient.** On the right side (Fig. 45) the deep cupping at the upper and lower margins of the optic disc are ophthalmoscopically strongly indicative of glaucoma. Nasally and temporally the excavation appears more shallow. One can recognize vessels bending over the superior and inferior margin of the optic disc and appearing again slightly displaced in the depth of the excavation. Repeated controls of the intraocular pressure, as well as perimetry showed no evidence of glaucoma, so that this is apparently a congenital anomaly in the sense of a rudimentary optic nerve coloboma. The temporal superior artery is varicose across the optic disc before its division. The circular atrophic crescent can be interpreted as due to the myopia (—6,5). It is segregated by a fine pigmented ring from the pale but otherwise normal fundus. On the left side (Fig. 46) the myopic crescent corresponds to the much higher myopia of —13,0. The oval optic disc is hardly cupped and is not sharply divided from its crescent.

**Fig. 47 and 48. Congenital retinal fold; right and left eye of the same 18-year-old patient.** On the right eye (Fig. 47) an arc-like fold is present temporal to the optic disc, and is in parts of balloon-like prominence and involving the macula area. On the left side (Fig. 48), one sees a sharply demarcated fold temporally in the middle periphery, which widens out as it reaches the ora. The eyes were otherwise normal. Vision on the right: hand movements directly in front of the eye; left: 5/25.
Contrary to other similar retinal lesions, e.g. retinoschisis, this condition was present at birth. The duplication of the retina stretches from the optic nerve disc to the lens and ciliary body respectively, and consists histologically of the inner retinal layers. The embryological cause of this malformation is not well understood. One assumes that this is a mesodermal abnormality, but not one of those combined with a persistent hyaloid artery. A haemorrhage in the membrana vasculosa lentis has also been suggested as a cause.

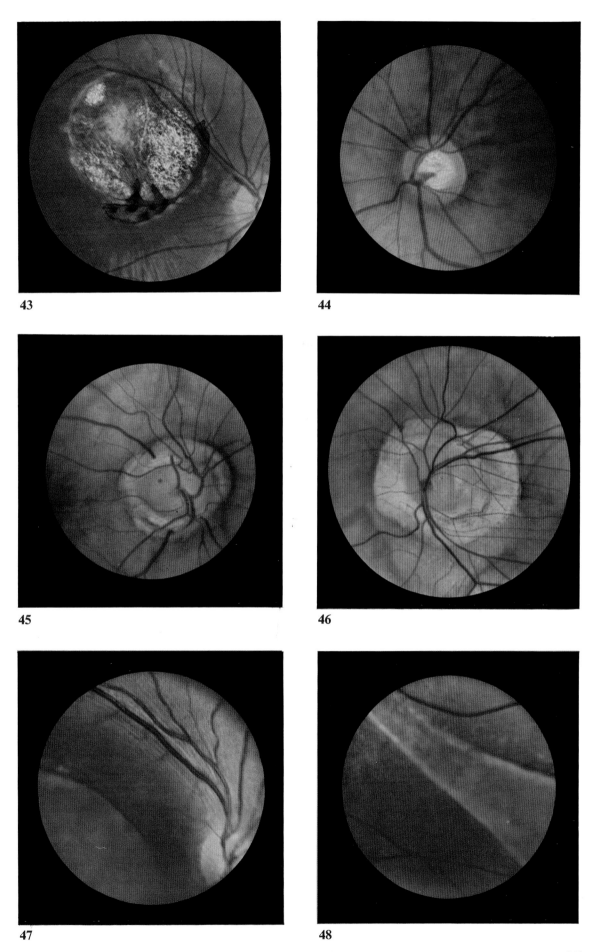

43

44

45

46

47

48

25

# Diseases of the optic nerve

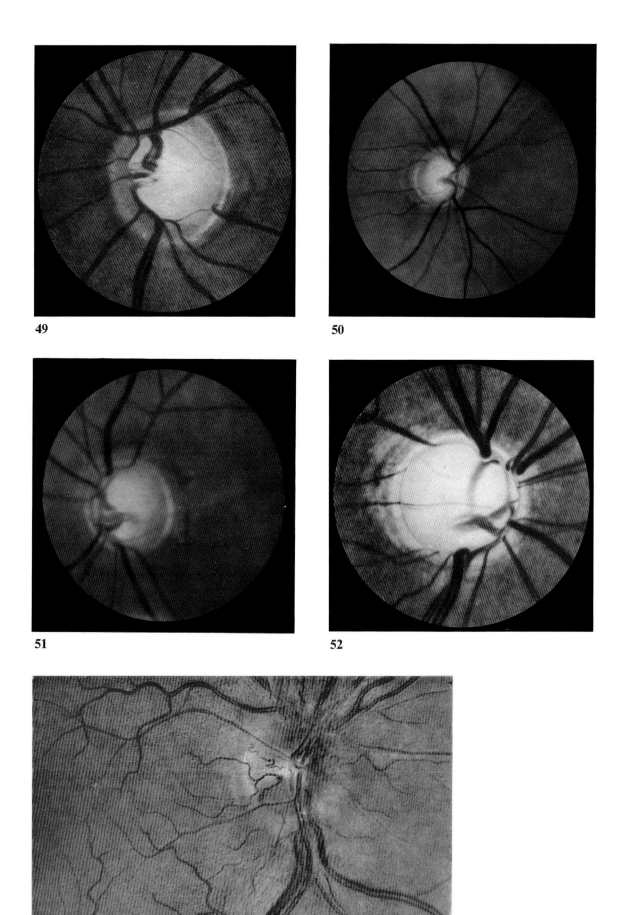

49

50

51

52

53

**Fig. 49. Onset of glaucomatous cupping; left eye.** The sclera is relatively weak where it is interrupted by the lamina cribrosa at the exit of the optic nerve fibres. Increased intraocular tension of lengthy duration leads to compression of capillaries here, which results in destruction of nerve fibres and thus to glaucomatous cupping. This cupping becomes progressively broader and deeper until it reaches the edge of the optic disc, so that the retinal vessels are nicked here, due to the difference in levels. In several cases the vascular tree is thus pushed nasally. This stage has just been reached in the picture shown. One can recognize almost complete cupping on the temporal side. At the base of the optic disc the markings of the lamina cribrosa are just visible.

**Fig. 50 and 51. Glaucomatous cupping; right and left eye (picture of left eye greatly enlarged).** Complete glaucomatous cupping on both sides, with an especially deep excavation of the optic disc reaching from the nasal to the temporal margin. The vascular tree is displaced nasally. Especially on the left side (Fig. 51) one can see the sharp bayonet-like bending of the larger veins. The difference in plane between the base of the optic disc and the retina is made visible by the course of the vessels. A chronic simple glaucoma was only recently discovered in this 71-year-old patient. Visual acuity: right 5/5, left 5/20, with extreme visual field defects on the left eye as well as on the right.

**Fig. 52. Glaucomatous atrophy of the optic disc; right eye.** If the intraocular tension remains abnormally high over a long period, the nerve fibres become atrophic and the cupped disc becomes greyish white and eventually completely pale. Here there is also a narrow glaucomatous halo around the optic disc.

**Fig. 53. Slight ischaemic papilloedema; right eye.** The nasal superior and inferior optic disc margins are blurred. Only the temporal margin remains sharply demarcated. No change in the arteries but considerable stasis on the venous side. The fact that this is a pathological change and not an anomaly is shown by the progression of the lesion. Visual acuity in this 56-year-old patient was at first 5/35–5/25 with a central scotoma. After treatment with vasodilators there was an improvement in visual acuity to 5/5.

**Fig. 54. Optic neuritis; left eye.** This 42-year-old patient suffered an inflammatory optic neuritis. There is blurring and slight prominence of the optic disc which has already turned somewhat pale. No constriction of the arteries and no congestion of the veins.

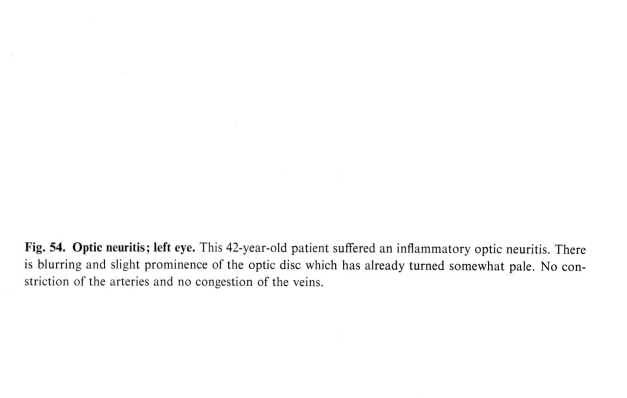

**Fig. 55–57. Optic neuritis; right eye.** 8 days after the onset of a decrease in visual acuity of unknown aetiology, one can see that the margins of the right optic disc are blurred on all sides (Fig. 55). The retinal veins are more varicose in some areas due to the stasis caused by the optic disc oedema. (The indistinct appearance of the photograph is due to vitreal opacities.) Figure 56 shows the same eye one week later. The vitreal opacities have receded. The state of the optic disc and its surroundings has remained unchanged except for a certain amount of increased venous stasis. A further 6 weeks later (Fig. 57) one can recognize a definite improvement: the temporal margin of the optic disc becomes more visible; the veil across the exit of the vessels has disappeared. There is now a return of normal visual acuity. The diminished venous stasis is another sign of the decreased oedema.

**Fig. 58. Considerable optic disc neuritis with secondary new vessel formation; left eye.** Here is the picture of an old inflammation of the optic disc which now shows new vessel formation and occasional dot and spot haemorrhages added to its blurred margins. There is also moderate varicosity and congestion of the dark veins. The arteries are slightly sheathed. In spite of intensive therapy this picture remained unaltered. The visual acuity remained low at 1/20 due to a centrocoecal scotoma.

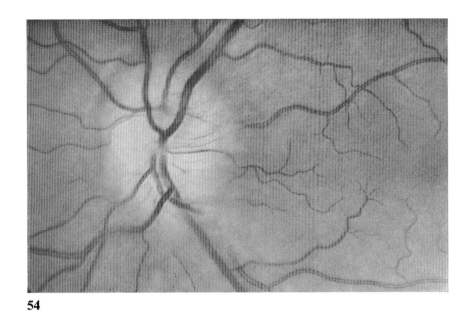

**54**

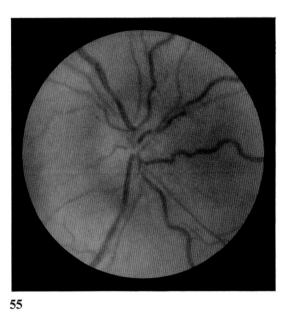

**55**

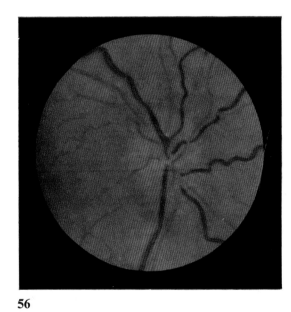

**56**

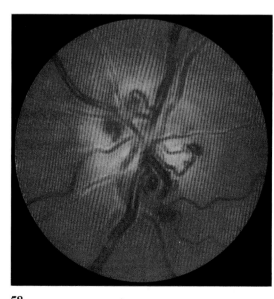

**57**

**58**

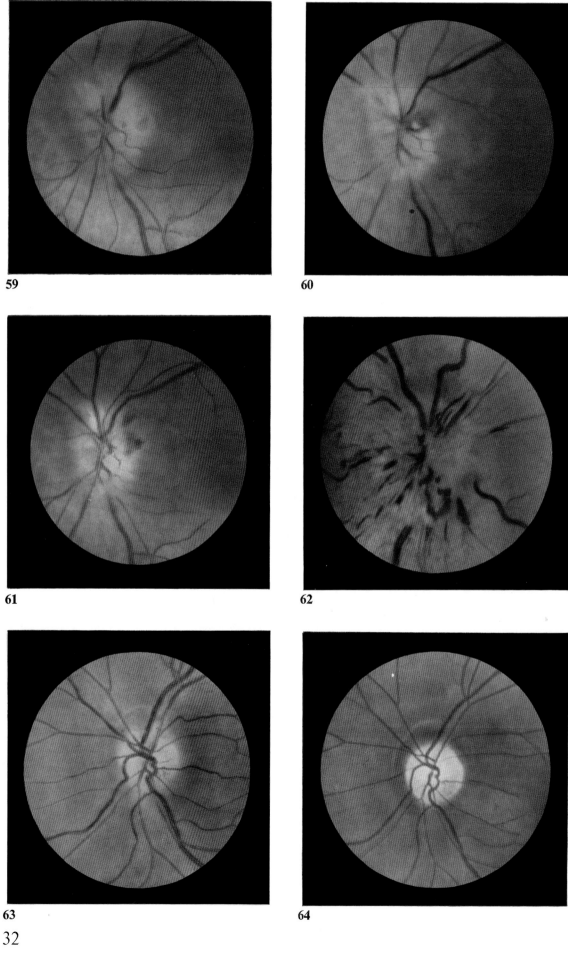

59

60

61

62

63

64

32

**Fig. 59–61. Vascular papilloedema; left eye.** The aetiology of the papilloedema was arteriosclerosis as shown by general examination. At first (Fig. 59) one saw a swelling and blurring of the optic disc with oedema and dot-shaped haemorrhages and a venous stasis of especially the temporal superior vein. 6 days later (Fig. 60) the oedematous area has become smaller. A diffuse haemorrhage at the temporal superior margin of the disc is a sign of the vascular damage. After 5 further days (Fig. 61) this haemorrhage has altered its form, while the other signs are unchanged. One can see signs of resorption, especially on further examinations. The margins of the optic disc have become more distinct.

**Fig. 62. Vascular papilloedema with hypertensive retinopathy; left eye.** The changes seen in the previous photographs are more extreme here. The optic disc is completely blurred and somewhat prominent on all sides but especially at its nasal inferior margin. The oedema encompasses the neighbouring retina, so that the exit of the large lower vascular branches has become partially invisible. There are several mainly longitudinal line-like haemorrhages and degenerative lesions. On the whole this is a picture of a papilloedema due to hypertensive changes (B.P. 205/115 mm Hg). This patient had suffered an apoplectic insult recently.

**Fig. 63 and 64. Optic neuritis with transition to atrophy; left eye.** This 30-year-old patient was admitted with a left-sided concentric visual field constriction with normal visual acuity. The optic disc (Fig. 63) was slightly blurred on all sides. There was slight venous stasis without haemorrhage. 29 days later (Fig. 64) an onset of optic disc atrophy was visible. The slight papilloedema and the venous stasis have disappeared. In spite of vaso-dilatory treatment, a sharply defined and distinctly pale optic disc is now visible. A general examination did not reveal an abnormality.

**Fig. 65. Onset of papilloedema; right eye.** The papilloedema is caused by an increase in intracranial pressure or a direct compression of the optic nerve. This results in a stasis of the venous branches of the circulation as well as the lymphatic channels in the optic nerve sheaths. The oedematous swelling of the scaffolding tissues of the nerve fibres, together with the purely mechanical factor, leads to a protuberance and blurring of the optic disc. Physiological cupping as in this case disappears. The oedema spreads in a varying degree into the retina, with stasis and increased varicosity of the retinal veins. Delicate streak haemorrhages are visible at the superior optic disc margin. The differentiation between a slight true papilloedema and an optic disc neuritis is not always possible ophthalmoscopically, but can be made by the examination of visual function. In optic neuritis there is a clinically rapid fall in visual acuity with a central scotoma; with true papilloedema the visual acuity is at least in the beginning normal (in our patient 5/4). The signs here were found by chance during examination of an out-patient who came because of a conjunctivitis.

**Fig. 66. Papilloedema; left eye.** One can see small dot and spot haemorrhages on the mushroom-like, swollen, 2 dptr-prominent, hyperaemic optic disc, over whose edge the retinal vessels course in the form of an arc. In the neighbourhood are irregular reflexes caused by the swelling of the retina and folding of Bruch's membrane. Neurological examination revealed signs of a left-sided cerebral process; further investigations were not possible due to domestic reasons.

**Fig. 67. Papilloedema; right eye of a 36-year-old patient.** This is the picture of a fresh papilloedema approximately 1½ dptr-prominent. The arteries are somewhat attenuated and the veins congested. In spite of the prominence of the optic disc the vessels are not submerged in the oedema. However the difference in levels can be recognized by the course of the vessels. Delicate haemorrhages are also present around the disc.

**Fig. 68. Older papilloedema; left eye of an 18-year-old.** This is the full picture of a massive, no longer fresh papilloedema of 5 dptr-prominence. One can now see white foci distributed across the whole optic disc region representing old haemorrhages which occurred at the onset of the disease. The vessels are partially obliterated by the oedema. The patient had a rapidly developing cerebellar tumour and died shortly after this examination.

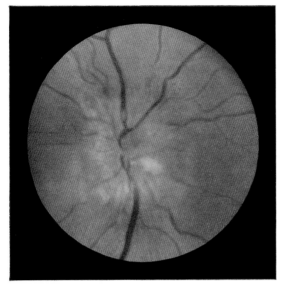

**65**

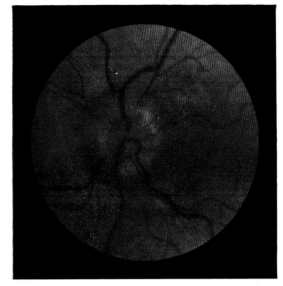

**66**

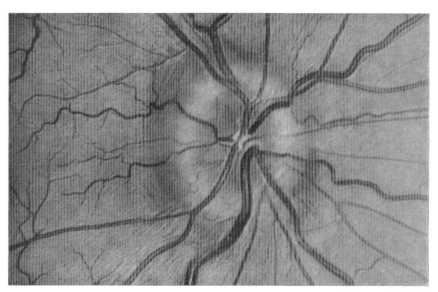

**67**

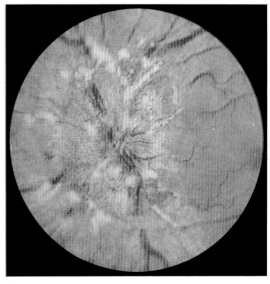

**68**

35

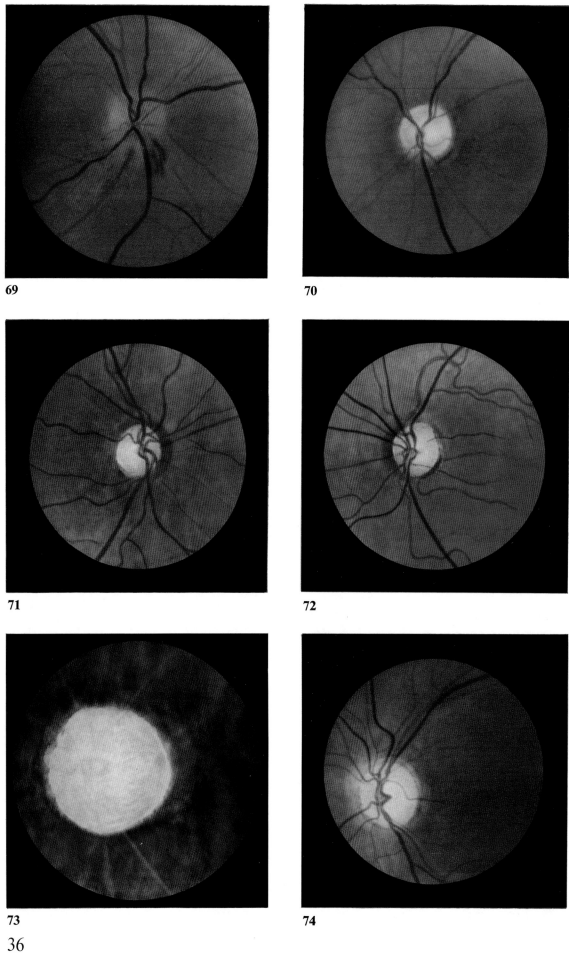

69

70

71

72

73

74

36

**Fig. 69 and 70. Foster Kennedy Syndrome (papilloedema of one optic disc, with simple atrophy of the other side); right and left eye of the same patient.** 75% of cases with papilloedema are due to a cerebral space-occupying lesion. The occurrence and the degree of the signs of stasis at the optic nerve head are dependent mostly on the site of the lesion. Thus for example, tumours of the Sylvian aquaduct or the foramen of Luschka and Magendi usually lead to early papilloedema; whereas, tumours at other sites must reach larger dimensions before they cause such signs. Tumours of the anterior cranial fossa, especially those of the frontal lobe, can occasionally cause a simple atrophy of the optic nerve on the side of the growth, due to direct compression, with papilloedema on the other side due to the disturbance in drainage. This 61-year-old patient with a papilloedema on the right side (Fig. 69) and the simple optic nerve atrophy on the left side (Fig. 70) had a left frontal lobe tumour, which manifested within a relatively short time, as is shown by the fresh signs of stasis on the right (haemorrhages at the inferior optic disc margin, Fig. 69) and by the only just-visible pallor of the optic disc (Fig. 70) with still almost normal vascular calibration.

**Fig. 71 and 72. Onset of simple optic nerve atrophy; right and left eye of the same patient.** The aetiology in this 28-year-old patient is a disseminated sclerosis which has been present for approx. 3 years. Irreversibly damaged optic nerves become pale. The pallid appearance of the optic disc here is also due to the clearly visible lamina cribrosa. Parallel to this change, but not so marked in this patient, is the narrowing of the retinal vessels. Every atrophy is naturally accompanied by a decrease in visual acuity, if not a complete amaurosis. The visual acuity in this patient was on the right 5/15, on the left 5/10.

**Fig. 73. Optic nerve atrophy; left eye. The optic nerve was severed due to a basal skull fracture 6 years ago, and was accompanied by sudden complete blindness.** Our greatly enlarged photograph shows a pale sharply demarcated optic disc lying in the plane of the retina with sharply defined markings of the lamina cribrosa. One can discern only occasional retinal vascular branches as narrow pale lines. Visual acuity on the right 5/5, the left eye is amaurotic. One must assume that the trauma to the optic nerve here included severing of the central artery as traumatic atrophies due to division of the optic nerve at the level of the optic canal (that is to say centrally from the entrance of the central artery into the optic nerve) do not usually cause such extreme changes of the retinal vessels.

**Fig. 74. Simple traumatic optic atrophy; left eye.** This 20-year-old patient suffered multiple skull fractures with sudden blindness on the left side following a fall from a motor scooter. After several weeks a simple atrophy developed here. In spite of the distinct narrowing of the vessels on the whole, the nasal section of the optic disc appears slightly more vascularized. – The electroretinogram has proved valuable in the differentiation between ascending (that is retinal), and descending optic atrophy. Ophthalmoscopically this differentiation is difficult. Ascending atrophy usually has an extinguished ERG; whereas, it is more or less well preserved in the descending atrophies.

**Fig. 75 and 76. Simple optic atrophy following arachnoiditis of the optic chiasm; right and left eye of the same patient.** This inflammation of the anterior basal skull damages the chiasm partially due to constrictive adhesions, and partly due to increased fluid pressure (via blockage of the ventricles). It does not cause typical changes in the visual fields. In the further course of the disease a simple optic atrophy can result as in our 22-year-old patient. Especially on the right eye (Fig. 75) one can see a definite pallor of the sharply defined optic disc, without definite vascular constriction. As a chance finding congenital venous tortuosity of some venous branches is also visible. Normal blood pressure. Visual acuity on the right is 5/7–5/5, on the left 5/10. Considerable concentric constriction of the right visual field, small central scotoma on the left.

**Fig. 77. Syphilitic optic atrophy; left eye.** Classical genuine descending optic atrophy in a 58-year-old man with tabes dorsalis. The pale optic disc lies in the same plane as the retina. The vessels are narrow. Visual acuity is perception of light with uncertain localisation.

**Fig. 78. Simple optic atrophy after radioactive-gold resection of the hypophyseal gland; right eye.** In this patient a tumour of the hypophyseal gland was treated with radioactive-gold implantation. Several months later, a decrease in visual acuity developed. Vision now includes only handmovements with uncertain light localisation on both sides. There is a pallor of the optic disc with dysversion, and a narrowing of the vessels entering and leaving the temporal optic disc margin respectively. There is broad nasal conus, and marked choroidal sclerosis,

**Fig. 79. Onset of temporal pallor after retrobulbar neuritis; right eye.** In this case repeated attacks of retrobulbar neuritis associated with a disseminated sclerosis took place. At first the optic disc was normal inspite of a central scotoma in the visual field. There is now however an onset of pallor temporally. Other changes are absent. The papillo-macular bundle of nerve fibres lying on the temporal side of the optic disc is more vulnerable than the rest of the optic nerve. The papillo-macular bundle constitutes a relatively large part of the total nerve fibres of the optic nerve when compared to the area of its supply, because in the area of the fovea and its immediate neighbourhood every receptor element of the retina possesses an individual central nervous connection (in the peripheral retina several photoreceptor cells are connected together to one nerve fibre). The temporal sector of the optic nerve disc is composed of the papillo-macular fibres. The visual field defect comprises the relatively small but functionally especially important centro-coecal area between the macula and the optic disc.

**Fig. 80. Onset of temporal pallor of the optic disc; right eye.** This 16-year-old patient has an already recognizable temporal pallor of the optic disc relating to a retrobulbar neuritis with disseminated sclerosis. The visual acuity was decreased to 5/10. This is an otherwise normal youthful reflex-rich fundus.

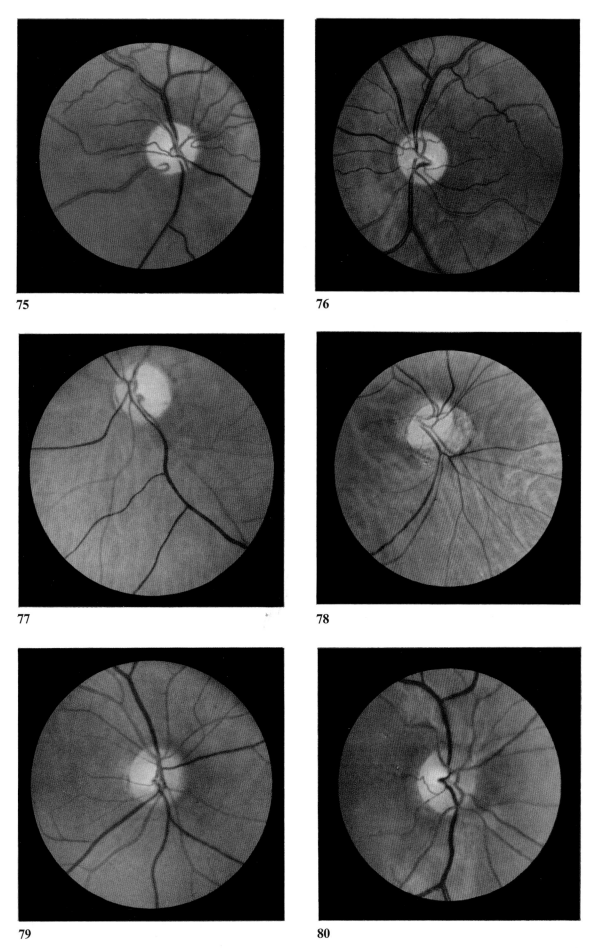

75

76

77

78

79

80

39

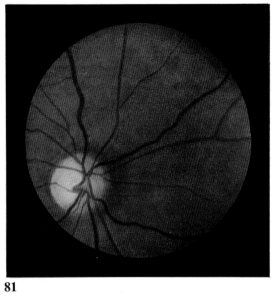

81

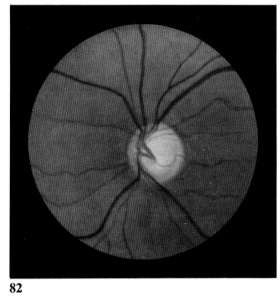

82

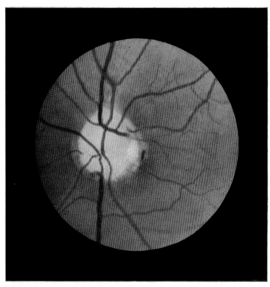

83

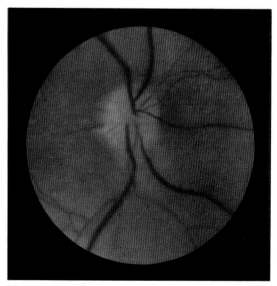

84

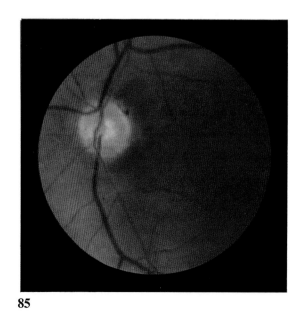

85

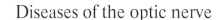

**Fig. 81 and 82. Temporal pallor of the optic disc; right and left eye of the same patient.** This 39-year-old patient has suffered from disseminated sclerosis since 3 years. The visual acuity in both eyes is 5/10. There is a marked pallor of the temporal half of the optic disc on both sides, with a large but not marginal physiological cupping, and with nicking of a small vessel. No glaucoma!

**Fig. 83. Postneuritic atrophy; left eye.** After papilloedema of long duration or after an optic neuritis, a postneuritic atrophy develops with blurred optic disc margins. Here is an altogether dirtyish pale-coloured optic disc with only its nasal superior margin sharply defined, and with the onset of vaso-constriction of the arterial branches, which demonstrates that this process began quite some time ago.

**Fig. 84 and 85. Postneuritic atrophy; right and left eye of the same 73-year-old patient.** Here the vascular changes of the retina must be interpreted as the substrate of a past vascular neuritis (accompanied by hypertension and arteriosclerosis). One can now recognize on the right side (Fig. 84) faint stellate exudate-like white areas of degeneration at the posterior pole between the macula lutea and the optic disc as a remnant of the previous oedema. The arteries especially on the left side are narrowed, with increased reflexes on the right. There is moderate venous stasis; whereas, one can still recognize the optic neuritis on the right eye; on the left (Fig. 85) a pallor of the blurred optic disc has begun to develop.

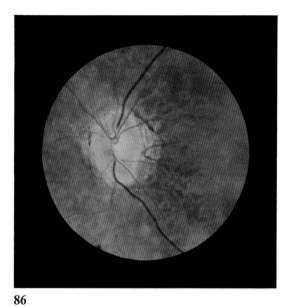

86

**Fig. 86. Waxy-yellow atrophy accompanying retinitis pigmentosa; left eye.** In the course of a disseminated tapeto-retinal degeneration of pigmentosa type (compare Fig. 234–246) an ascending optic atrophy occurs, similar to that after central arterial occlusion. This is characterized by a waxy-yellow colour and often slightly indistinct margins of the optic disc. The marked attenuation of the vessels, especially of the arteries, and the sclerotic choroidal vessels are clearly visible.

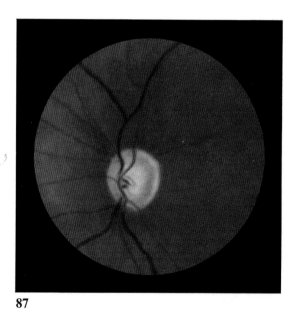

87

**Fig. 87. Retinal atrophy after central arterial occlusion; left eye.** This 20-year-old patient suffered from endocarditis, which probably resulted in the retinal vascular occlusion due to emboli of the in-flammatory encrustations on the cardiac valves. Here are findings 8 weeks after occlusion of the central retinal artery. The optic disc is pale yellow and sharply defined, with constricted vessels. Visual acuity: amaurosis.

# Diseases of the retina

## Vascular lesions

# Diseases of the retina

**Fig. 88 and 89. Central retinal arterial occlusion; right eye.** It has been proved that so-called embolic occlusion of the central artery results more often from hypertensive and (or) sclerotic changes of the vascular wall, rather than from true emboli. Vascular spasm probably plays a part. According to most authors however, the latter does not generally lead to a complete and irreversible interruption of bloodflow. The picture (Fig. 88) here shows the retina of a 46-year-old hypertensive patient taken 18 hours after onset of the vascular occlusion. Due to the ischaemic oedema of the retina, the whole fundus is pale with somewhat narrowed arteries. At the posterior pole the fovea stands out in contrast as a cherry-red spot, due to the choroid glimmering through the retina. 20 days later (Fig. 89), the retinal oedema has been almost completely resorbed. The fundus has almost a normal colour; the cherry-red spot is only faintly visible, the retinal arteries are constricted. A waxy-yellow optic atrophy developed later. In spite of intensive treatment with vasodilators, visual acuity could only be improved to a level of hand-movements in 1 m.

**Fig. 90. Occlusion of a cilio-retinal artery; 43-year-old patient, right eye.** The oedema in branch occlusion is confined to the area of supply of the vessel involved. If as in this case a cilio-retinal artery supplies the area of sharpest vision, then there appears as in central arterial occlusion, a cherry-red spot at the centre of the oedematous zone. The occluded cilio-retinal artery which divides fork-like around the macula is constricted and surrounded by a pale oedematous halo. Visual acuity was hand-movements directly in front of the eye, with a large central scotoma.

**Fig. 91. Occlusion of the temporal inferior artery in diabetes; right eye.** This 56-year-old patient had suffered from diabetes mellitus since 6 years. During an ophthalmological examination a sudden arterial branch occlusion occurred with a decrease in visual acuity to 1/35 seen eccentrically. He was admitted immediately and treated with fibrinolysin. Thereupon, an improvement in visual acuity to 0,6 occurred. The ischaemic oedema visible temporal to the optic disc in the picture here, disappeared after 3 days.

**Fig. 92 and 93. Arterial branch occlusion due to sclerotic changes; right and left eye.** This 64-year-old patient suffered from occasional slight hypertension and extreme arteriosclerosis (at the time the photograph was taken B.P 145/110 mm Hg). Just before this, he had suffered sudden decrease in vision on the right eye. The picture (Fig. 92) shows the site of occlusion of the superior temporal narrowed artery to be in the optic nerve. The other arteries are also somewhat attenuated. Further signs that the optic nerve is involved, are the indistinct margins of the optic disc with slight prominence, oedema and a few haemorrhages. On the left (Fig. 93) is an occlusion of a superior arterial branch from a few months previously, which has reversed almost completely. Remarkable is, however, the stasis and varicosity of the veins on both sides. Visual acuity: right 5/50; left 5/5.

44

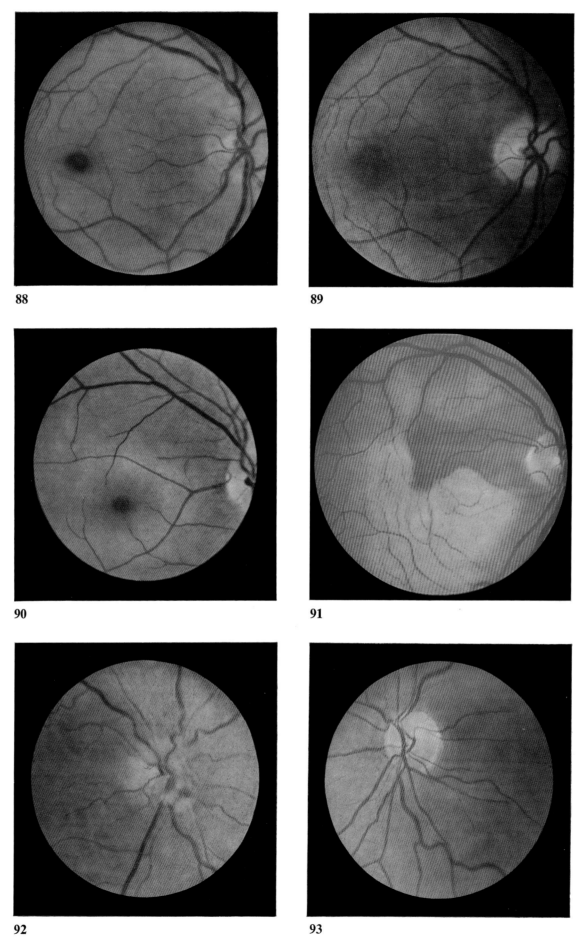

88

89

90

91

92

93

45

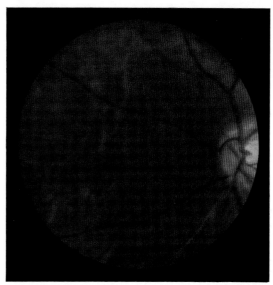

**94**

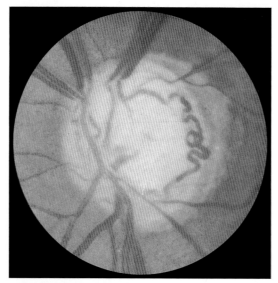

**95**

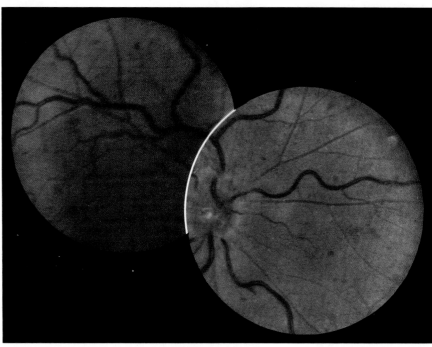

**96**

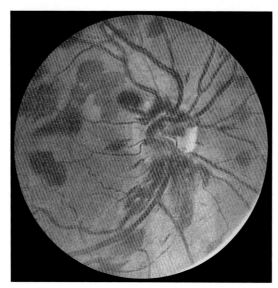

**97**

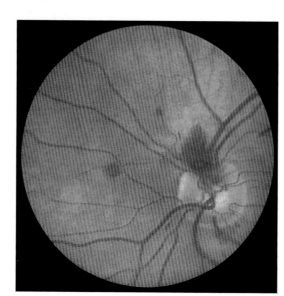

**98**

**Fig. 94. Fundus after occlusion of the nasal inferior artery; right eye.** This shows that an arterial branch occlusion can occur on the basis of sclerotic changes. This only just 48-year-old patient also suffered from extreme arteriosclerosis of the cerebral vessels. In the picture one can see the nasal inferior arterial branch obliterated for approx. a year, and now visible as a white strand devoid of blood. There is also extreme choroidal sclerosis.

**Fig. 95. Venous rete mirabile on the optic disc; left eye.** This 69-year-old patient suffered from glaucoma since 2 years, which remained decompensated in spite of treatment with miotics and carbonic anhydrase inhibitors (Diamox®). The patient refused surgery. Visual acuity was normal. Visual field examination showed a round subcentral scotoma without a connection to the blind spot. A new vessel can be seen running corkscrew-like at the temporal margin of the optic disc cup. This is the result of an old central retinal vein thrombosis.

**Fig. 96. So-called prethrombosis of the central retinal vein; right eye.** This 75-year-old hypertensive patient (B.P. 190/115 mm Hg) had a visual acuity of 5/5–5/4. Foremost in the picture is the stasis and the increased varicosity of the venous branches. Delicate dot and spot haemorrhages can be seen everywhere, as well as the onset of slight optic disc prominence with blurring of the margins. The nasal inferior vein disappears shortly before its entrance into the oedematous optic disc margin. The haemorrhages as well as the optic disc changes disappeared practically completely under an anticoagulative treatment with coumarine (Marcumar®).

**Fig. 97. Incomplete occlusion of the central retinal vein; right eye.** The fundus of this 56-year-old patient shows large round and stripe haemorrhages especially around the area of the optic disc, but also reaching the macula with an otherwise almost normal vascular pattern. The general circulation was normal. The patient suffered from a metastasising mammary carcinoma, however, without ocular or cerebral metastasis.

**Fig. 98. Incomplete central retinal vein occlusion; right eye.** This is a picture of the same patient shown in Fig. 97, one year and four months later. The haemorrhages have been mostly resorbed. There is still a large haemorrhage present near the optic disc, surrounded by smaller dot and stripe haemorrhages. Degenerative foci have not yet developed.

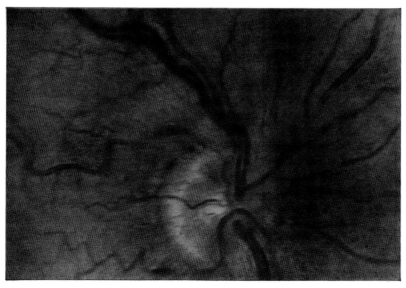

**99**

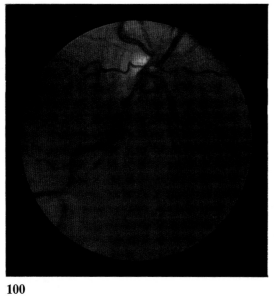

**100**

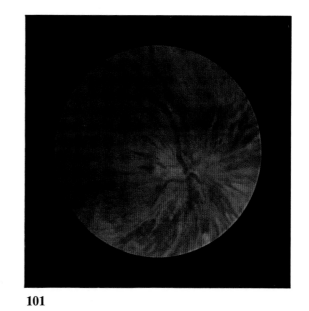

**101**

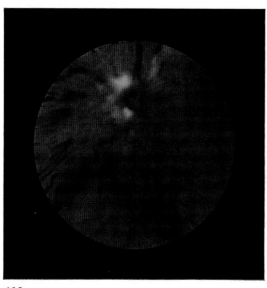

**102**

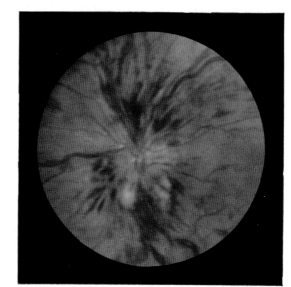

**103**

**Fig. 99. Threatening central venous occlusion; right eye.** This only just 41-year-old patient (B.P. 160/100 mm Hg) has typical signs of hypertensive retinopathy as this somewhat enlarged picture shows: irregular vascular calibration, dark colouring and increased varicosity of the temporal superior vein with a faint Gunn's sign at the superior papillary margin, onset of arterial constriction, an already quite blurred optic disc margin with increased nerve-fibre markings especially nasally, and prominently visible hyperaemic capilleries on the optic disc. The eye still had full visual acuity.

**Fig. 100. "Prethrombosis" of the central retinal vein with hypertension; right eye.** Here a central retinal venous occlusion occured 4 months later. – One sees a dark red fundus with stasis and irregular calibration of the retinal venous branches and marked constriction of the arteries with broad reflexes. The optic disc is blurred at its inferior margin. The temporal inferior vein is somewhat veiled by the onset of the optic disc oedema in this sector.

**Fig. 101. Fresh "thrombosis" of the central retinal vein; right eye.** Full picture of a central retinal vein occlusion with massive haemorrhages. The optic disc is completely blurred and surrounded by mostly radially placed haemorrhages. The rest of the fundus including the periphery also has haemorrhages of varying size, form and density, mostly covering the vessels. The appearance of the haemorrhages relates to their topography within the retina: pale surface haemorrhages = preretinal location; flame-shaped radial haemorrhages = nerve fibre layer; dot and spot haemorrhages = nuclear layers. If the centre of the retina is affected as here, the visual acuity can be very much reduced. Generally however central retinal venous occlusion contrary to central retinal arterial occlusion is compatible with more or less good vision. As is now recognized, the occlusion of the central retinal vein is not necessarily due to a true thrombosis. Sclerotic changes of the vascular wall play an important part among other factors. This 50-year-old patient had a blood pressure of 180/110 mm Hg.

**Fig. 102. Central retinal vein occlusion; left eye.** Here especially one can see radial haemorrhages arranged according to the nerve fibre layer in which they are located. The optic disc margins are completely obliterated; the vessels in the region of the optic disc hardly visible.

**Fig. 103. Central retinal venous (not quite fresh) occlusion; left eye.** This state has been present since 2½ months. One sees a slightly prominent circularly blurred and hyperaemic optic disc, with numerous large and small spot haemorrhages, which are especially numerous around the optic disc and become more scant towards the periphery. At the inferior margin of the optic disc are several yellowish white degenerative areas, which indicate that the onset of the disease was some time ago. There is engorgement and increased varicosity of the retinal veins. Investigations in recent years have shown that central retinal venous occlusion occurring in young otherwise apparently healthy individuals presents especially when the blood pressure is abnormally low. This 38-year-old patient's blood pressure was 115/75 mm Hg.

**Fig. 104. Occlusion of a small retinal venous branch; right eye.** If as here only a small vascular branch is occluded, then principally the same signs occur as in central retinal venous occlusion only now confined to a circumscribed area. Venous branch occlusions often take place at the site of an arterial-venous crossing. Here one sees haemorrhages above the superior temporal vein just before its entrance into the optic disc, due to occlusion of a small vein in this area. Changes of this nature are usually not noticed by the patient. The dark colouring and slight dilation of the retinal veins constitute slight signs of hypertension.

**Fig. 105. Occlusion of a temporal inferior venous branch; right eye.** In this 70-year-old patient a small vessel reaches the macula region from below. An occlusion occurring 28 days previously led to pre- as well as intraretinal cockade-like haemorrhages, which surround a pale degenerative area. At its temporal edge the haemorrhage shows the radial striping corresponding to the retinal nerve-fibre layer. This haemorrhage led to a decrease in visual acuity to 5/15. After its resorption delicately pigmented areas remained in the macula. The visual acuity was now 5/7.

**Fig. 106. Fresh occlusion of the inferior venous branches; left eye.** In the area of supply of the occluded veins, i.e. the inferior half of the fundus, spot and flame-shaped haemorrhages encompass the macula from below. Numerous haemorrhages also lie on the indistinctly bordered optic disc. Degenerative areas are still absent, as the occlusion occurred only recently.

**Fig. 107. Older occlusion of practically the whole temporal inferior venous branch; right eye.** This 50-year-old patient suffered from hypertension since 15 years. Blood pressure was now 210/110 mm Hg. 6 weeks ago there occurred a decrease in visual acuity on the right eye to 5/10. There is extreme engorgement and irregular calibration of the temporal inferior vein practically up to its entrance at the optic disc. In its peripheral area of supply there are massive, mostly spot haemorrhages. Cotton-wool-like degenerative areas, as well as the faintly visible stellate exudates between the optic disc and the macula, indicate the longstanding presence of a circulatory disorder.

**Fig. 108. Not-quite-fresh occlusion of the inferior temporal vein; left eye.** This 74-year-old patient with arteriosclerosis and hypertension (B.P. 250/130 mm Hg) had an onset of "branch venous thrombosis" 3 weeks ago. The occluded vein is only visible just before its entrance into the optic disc. In the foreground are massive haemorrhages in the area of the temporal inferior vascular arc, which have in places encompassed the optic disc. Yellow-white degenerative areas lie in between.

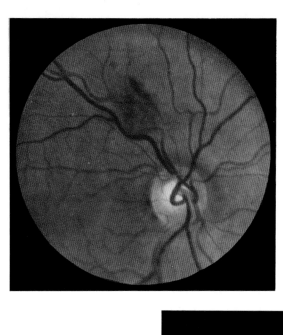

104

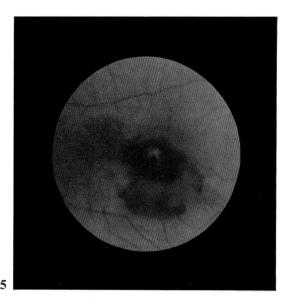

105

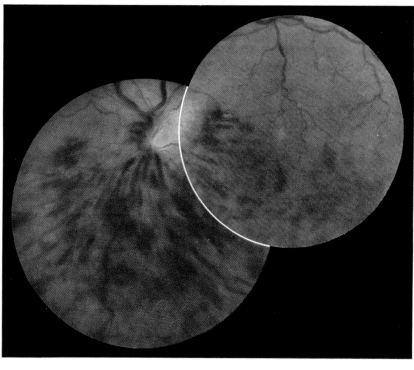

106

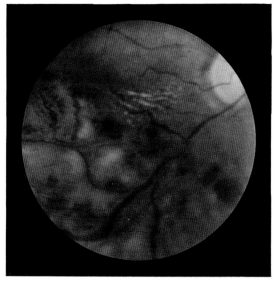

107

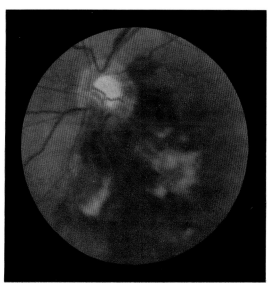

108

**Fig. 109. Older venous branch occlusion; left eye.** The temporal superior vein is occluded. The haemorrhages are comparatively scant in this case, so that the occluded, varicosed, and irregularly-calibrated, engorged vessel with its branches although indistinct remains visible practically along its whole course. Signs of resorption in the form of degenerative areas and the onset of pigmentation, indicate that the occlusion occured several weeks ago.

**Fig. 110. Incomplete occlusion of several venous branches in hypertensive retinopathy grade III; right eye.** The engorgement, and in places increased varicosity of the inferior temporal vein and a small venous branch lying between the optic disc and the macula, as well as the attenuated arteries point to the underlying disease. Flame-shaped and dot haemorrhages lie in the area of supply of the inferior temporal vein, as well as at the superior temporal optic disc margin. The macula is the site of stellate exudate-like degenerative areas. Similar lesions in the form of a developing "retinitis circinata" are just below the centre of the retina.

**Fig. 111. The same fundus 4 weeks later.** Whereas the vessels remained unchanged in their general appearance, the stellate exudate-like degenerative areas at the posterior pole have increased in intensity and in size. Just beneath the optic disc is a now large flame-shaped haemorrhage lying almost completely preretinally. Fresh smaller haemorrhages have occurred directly above and along the inferior temporal vein, whereas others have been resorbed.

**Fig. 112. Old venous branch occlusion; right eye.** Due to the occlusion of the temporal superior vein a wide-spread collateral circulation has developed. The previous haemorrhages have been almost completely resorbed.

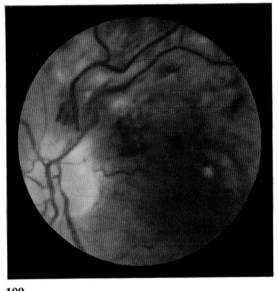

**109**

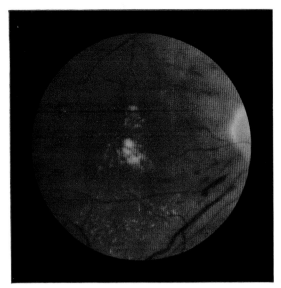

**110**

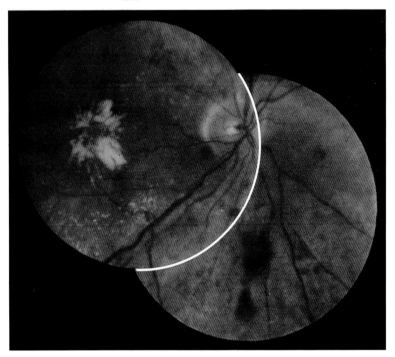

**111**

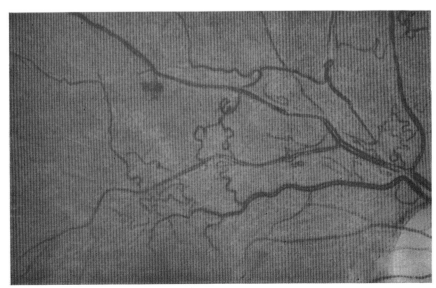

**112**

53

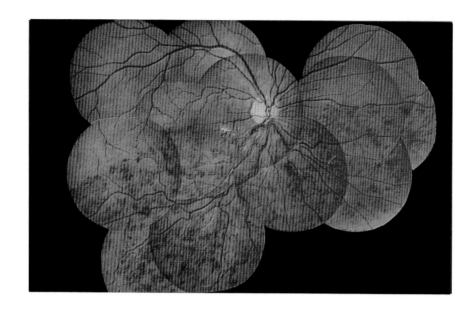

**113**

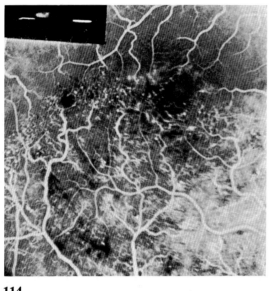

**114**

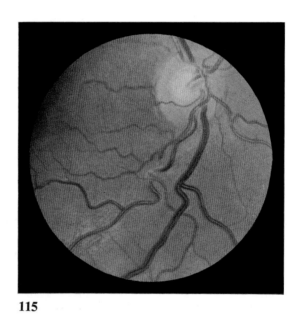

**115**

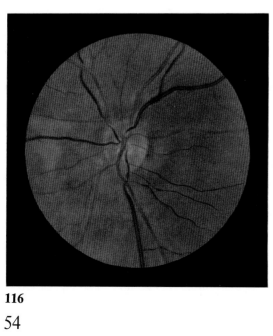

**116**

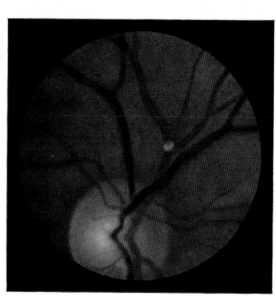

**117**

**Fig. 113. Venous branch occlusion; right eye.** This 61-year-old patient noticed a dark cloud in his right eye about a year ago. An occlusion of an inferior venous branch was discovered a few weeks later seen in the present picture. Anticoagulative therapy brought no improvement.

**Fig. 114. Fluorescenceangiography in venous branch occlusion; right eye.** The fluorescenceangiography of the fundus in Fig. 113 shows innumerable small leakages in the macula region as a sign of inadequate circulation in the region of the occluded vessel. Visual acuity was reduced to 0,6–0,8. Treatment with Argon-laser-coagulation resulted in an improvement in visual acuity to 1,0.

**Fig. 115. Hypertensive retinopathy; right eye.** Engorgement of the veins with somewhat broad reflexes. At the first fork of the temporal inferior artery is a small cotton-wool focus. The smaller vessels are slightly varicose. This 30-year-old patient has had moderate hypertension for 2½ years.

**Fig. 116. Hypertensive vascular changes; left eye.** Note moderate narrowing and stretched course of the arterial branches, with broad axial reflexes and irregularities in venous calibre. Also note distinct compression-signs of Gunn, nasally superior to the optic disc. According to Thiel's classification, which has proved valuable, this picture would correspond to stage I–II. As has been shown recently, Gunn's sign cannot be regarded simply as a circumscribed compression of the vein by the crossing artery. Certain investigations indicate that these crossing phenomena are caused as a rule by changes in the vascular wall, in the sense of increased thickness and density of the perivascular sheaths. Hypertrophied and proliferated glial and adventitial tissues are apparently much less transparent than the nerve fibre tissue which usually occurs at this site.

**Fig. 117. Moderate degree of hypertensive retinopathy; right eye.** Engorgement of the venous branches with slight irregularity in the calibre of the veins and arteries. The first fork of the superior temporal artery is the site of a so-called plaque, a similar lesion lies temporally inferiorly at a small arterial branch just before the exit from the optic disc. One finds these plaques especially at arterial bifurcation. Not infrequently they correspond to the site of a future arterial vascular occlusion. However one must not regard them as the most visible precursor of an embolus; because firstly, they can be larger than the vascular lumen, and secondly, they can occasionally decrease in size as repeated examinations have shown. Today one tends to regard plaques rather as representing reflex phenomena than as proliferative changes of the vascular wall.

**Fig. 118. Fundus changes in transitional hypertension; left eye.** This 53-year-old patient suffered from hypertension since at least 5 years. The enlarged photograph shows a plaque in the region of the arterial bifurcation, just after the first crossing of the temporal superior artery over the vein. The nature of these plaque formations as reflexes or mural changes respectively, is shown clearly in the upper right part of the picture: here one sees cuff-like sheathing interrupted centrally, of a superior branch of the artery after a further bifurcation. Otherwise there are increased gold-yellow arterial reflexes (copper-wire arteries), a Gunn's sign and a Salus' sign. The latter is an arc-like deflection of a vein directly under an artery.

**Fig. 119 and 120. Hypertensive and sclerotic changes; right and left eye of the same 71-year-old patient.** Right eye (Fig. 119): in the periphery as well as near the optic disc are several sites where fine flame and spot haemorrhages have occurred. Several Gunn's signs are faintly visible. Yellow-white degenerative areas in the region of the macula as well as the increased sclerotic tabulation of the choroid are an expression of the accompanying sclerotic circulatory disorder. Left eye (Fig. 120): here there are principally the same changes. Remarkable is the temporal inferior vascular arc: directly after the artery crosses over the vein, the venous branch coursing superiorly shows a hairpin-like bend (early venous branch occlusion?). Inferior to this are small spot haemorrhages with striped sclerotic depigmentation.

**Fig. 121. Fundus in transitional hypertension; left eye.** This 58-year-old patient had blood pressure values up to 230/150 mm Hg. Note the constriction of the arteries, engorgement and irregular calibration of the veins. Especially noticeable is the cotton-wool "exudate" situated near the temporal superior optic disc margin. This is a yellowish white, dull, cotton-wool-like lesion which represents ischaemic swelling of nerve-fibre axons in the area of supply of a non-functioning capillary.

56

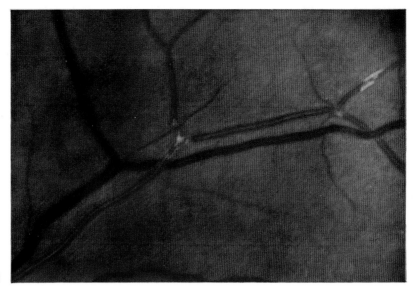

118

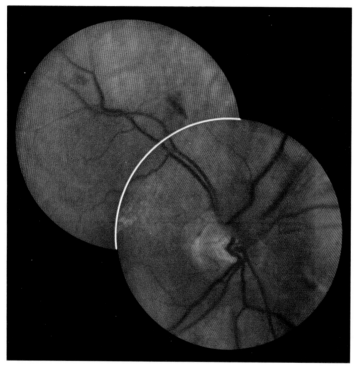

119

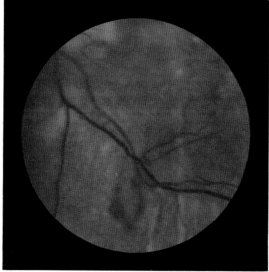

120

121

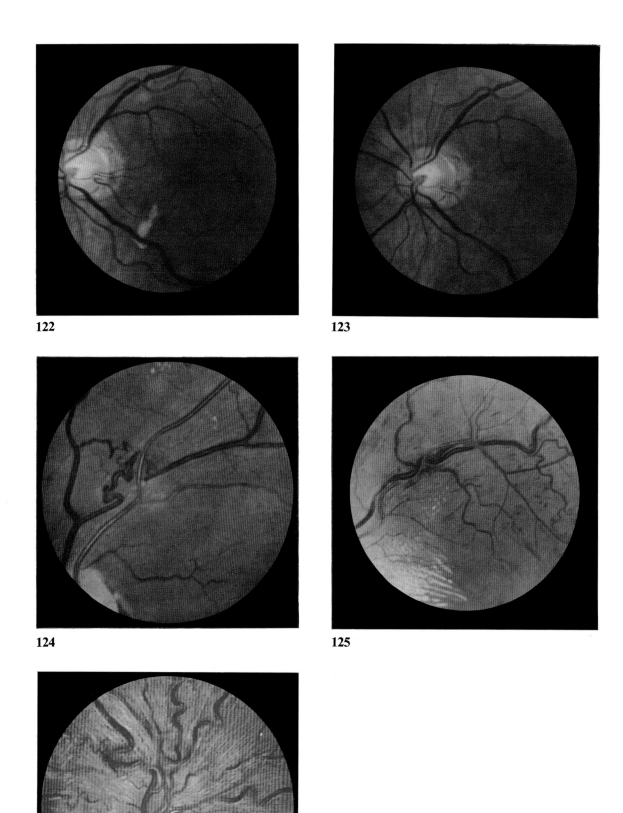

122

123

124

125

126

58

**Fig. 122 and 123. Fundus in transitional hypertension; left eye.** Hypertension was discovered ¾ of a year ago in this 38-year-old patient (B.P. 240/110 mm Hg). In addition to the engorgement and irregular calibration of the veins, narrowed arteries, and distinct signs of compression at the temporal superior vascular arc, one can recognize some distance temporal and inferior to the optic disc a cotton-wool lesion, over which an apparently uninvolved temporal inferior vein crosses. In addition there is a narrow (myopic) temporal crescent. 6 months later (Fig. 123), the engorgement of the veins has decreased and the cotton-wool focus has disappeared after antihypertensive treatment. In contrast to this one can still see haemorrhages in the periphery.

**Fig. 124. Rete mirabile-like vascular anastomosis; left eye.** This 60-year-old patient has suffered from hypertension since approx. 28 years. A distinct sign of Gunn was seen earlier in the temporal superior area of the fundus. A venous branch occlusion occurred here years ago. In the ensuing time this markedly varicosed vessel has developed, stretching over the interrupted section of the vein. The occasional white degenerative lesions in the area of supply of the temporal superior venous branch represent further remnants of the venous occlusion. Added to this are the broad axial reflexes of the otherwise attenuated arteries.

**Fig. 125. Fundus in renal hypertension; left eye.** Massive constriction of the arteries with broad light axial reflexes (silver-wire arteries). Engorgement and increased vascularity of the veins with marked signs of Gunn. In the region of the superior temporal vein are innumerable spot and flame-shaped haemorrhages, with occasional delicate pale foci. Between the optic disc and the macula is a stellate-exudate degeneration which corresponds to the nerve fibre radiations in this area. These fundus changes in this 51-year-old patient were even more marked 1½ years later.

**Fig. 126. Angiospastic retinopathy; right eye.** This 12-year-old girl suffered from hypertension since the second year of life with practically nonfunctioning kidneys so that haemodialysis was necessary. Visual acuity on both sides was reduced to 0,7. The blurred optic disc with oedema, the varicosed tortuous veins, and the extreme attenuation of the arteries are signs of the advanced hypertension.

**Fig. 127. Angiospastic retinopathy; right eye.** This 31-year-old patient had a blood pressure reading of 235/160 mm Hg. In the foreground is the onset of the optic disc blurring, the extreme spastic narrowing of the arteries which are hardly visible in places, the venous stasis as well as several cotton-wool ischaemic infarctions and fine stripe and dot haemorrhages.

**Fig. 128 and 129. Angiospastic retinopathy; right and left eye of the same 41-year-old patient.** Both optic discs are blurred especially nasally. Extreme, partially thread-like constriction of the arteries. The vessels are partially obscured by the peripapillery oedema. On both sides the macula has a stellate exudative degeneration. Next to this are numerous dot-spot and flame-shaped haemorrhages, as well as several cotton-wool "exudates". On the left eye (Fig. 129) directly superior to the optic disc, is an occlusion of a small venous branch. Nasally in the periphery is an aberrant bundle of myelinated nerve fibres (compare Fig. 28–30) as an accessory finding. Remarkably enough there are occasional dot haemorrhages also within this bundle.

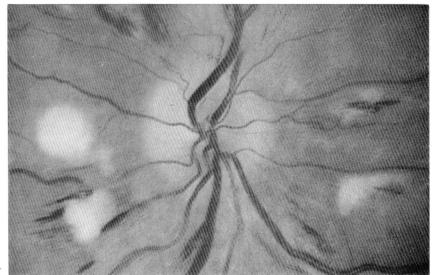

127

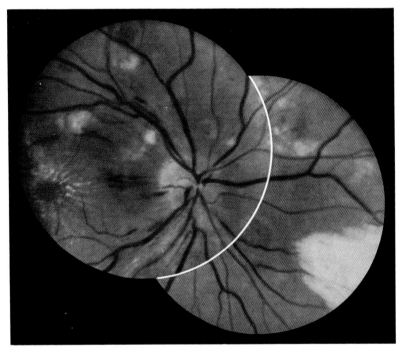

128

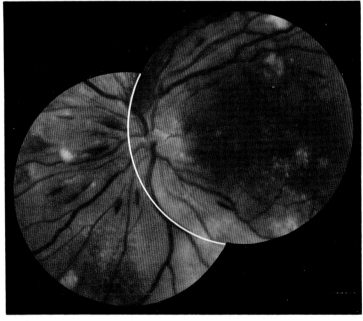

129

61

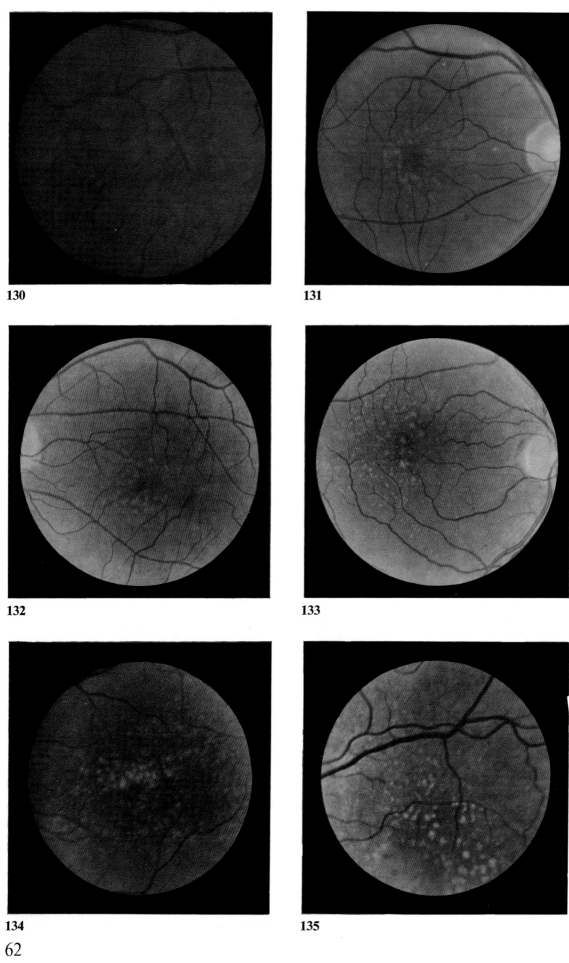

130

131

132

133

134

135

62

**Fig. 130. Simple arteriosclerotic fundus; left eye.** There are no functional defects in a simple arterio-sclerotic fundus. There is a diminished circulation corresponding to the size of the retinal vessels. The central fundus now poor in reflexes has achieved a "dull" appearance in this 47-year-old patient.

**Fig. 131 and 132. Simple arteriosclerotic fundus; right and left eye of the same 68-year-old patient.** Here delicate, bright dot-like foci have occurred in the region of the macula as a further sign of a simple arterio-sclerotic fundus. They are confluent in some places. Added to this, is the slightly increased varicosity of some of the smaller paramacular vessels. Visual acuity was normal.

**Fig. 133. Transition between simple arteriosclerotic fundus and the dry form of arteriosclerotic chorio-retinopathy; right eye.** The dry form of arteriosclerotic chorioretinopathy presents as hyperpigmented and depigmented areas of varying size, form and location. Small spot-like depigmentations in the central area of the fundus dominate in this case. These dysoric signs define the picture. The dry atrophic (senile) macula degeneration develops in the centre of the fundus, with a central scotoma, and therefore with a more or less decreased visual acuity.

**Fig. 134. Dry form of arteriosclerotic chorioretinopathy; left eye.** The dysoric, pale, mainly small-spotted foci are closer together here, and cover a larger area as in the case above. In the centre of the fundus they unite to somewhat larger lesions. In between are faintly visible pigmented borders. Visual acuity was 5/15 in this 54-year-old patient.

**Fig. 135. Dry form of arteriosclerotic chorioretinopathy; left eye.** In the foreground are sharply de-marcated, somewhat irregularly formed dysoric foci, which diminish in size toward the periphery. Sometimes they appear very close to small vascular branches. They commence here only at the margin of the macula. The fundus is reflexless and with moderate varicosity of the retinal venules.

**Fig. 136 and 137. Dry form of arteriosclerotic chorioretinopathy; right and left eye of the same 60-year-old patient.** The dysoric pale foci are not always confined to the central fundus. Occasionally as here, they can be seen far out in the periphery. Remarkable is the varying size of the foci, which sometimes unite to form broad plaques. Superior to the reflexless right macula (Fig. 136), is a glittering cholesterol focus with fine pigmentary changes directly inferior to it. The retinal vessels do not appear changed. These findings were at first misdiagnosed as a disseminated tapeto-retinal degeneration of pigmentosa type, because of the diffuse distribution of the pale foci. The electroretinogram, the peripheral visual fields and the dark-adaptation curve were however normal.

**Fig. 138. Dry form of arteriosclerotic chorioretinopathy; right eye.** Here glittering cholesterol deposits are especially visible at the central fundus. A broad belt-like pale area consisting of dysoric foci of varying size surrounds this zone. The findings in the other eye were analogous. Visual acuity in this 49-year-old patient was right 5/5, left 5/10–5/7; serum lipid content was normal.

**Fig. 139 and 140. Dry (right) and developing wet (left) arteriosclerotic macula degeneration.** Remarkable in this 56-year-old patient is the disappearance of the precapillaries on both sides. The macula area appears especially avascular. Between the extremely small dysoric foci right (Fig. 139) are irregular delicate pigment accumulations. On the left (Fig. 140), one can see a polymorphous depigmented focus lying in the plane of the retina in the region of the macula with an increased pigmented centre and a border. This zone is surrounded by a belt of dysoric foci of varying size which approx. reach the equator. Visual acuity: right 5/20, left 5/35; central scotoma.

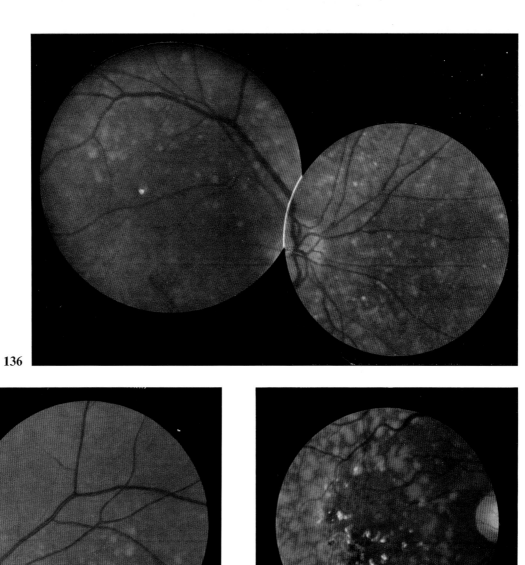

136

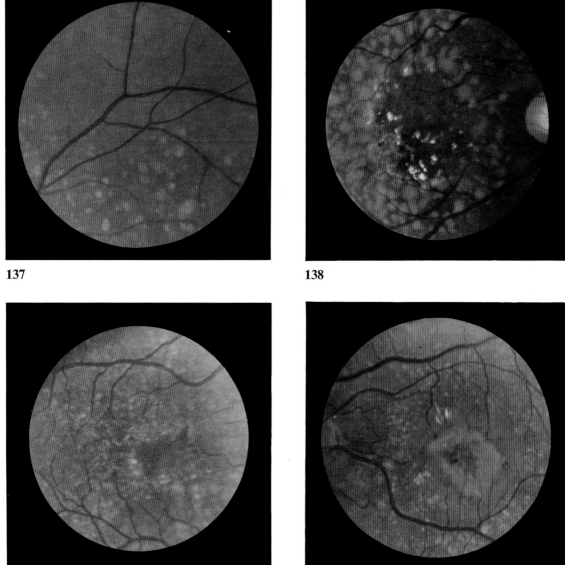

137

138

139

140

65

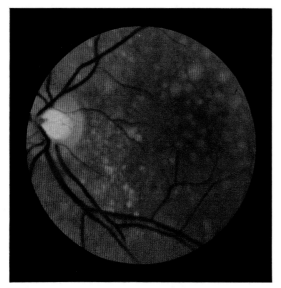

**141**

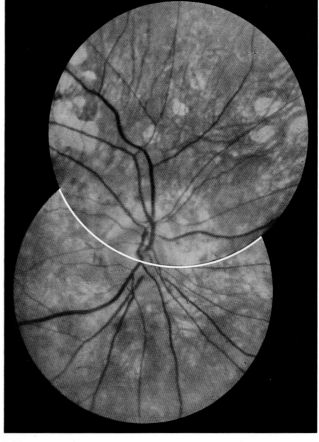

**142**

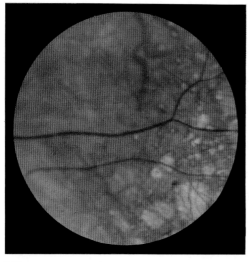

**143**

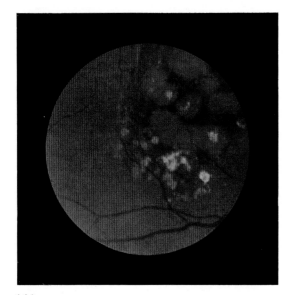

**144**

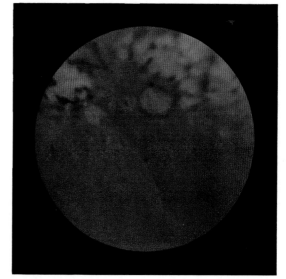

**145**

**Fig. 141. Dry form of arteriosclerotic chorioretinopathy; left eye.** In this case, the varying size of the pale foci are noticeable. They spread from the optic disc to the equator and beyond. In and superior to the reflexless macula, the foci remind one in form and diameter of drusen. Delicate pigmentary changes at the centre of the fundus.

**Fig. 142. Dry form of arteriosclerotic chorioretinopathy; right eye.** The large pale areas also dominate in this 58-year-old patient but contrary to the previous case, they especially encompass the central fundus. The peripapillary area is particularly affected, so that the rarification of the choroid reminds one of a myopic atrophy. The eye is emmetropic, however.

**Fig. 143. Dry form of arteriosclerotic chorioretinopathy; right eye.** Occasionally the changes are confined to the periphery, as in this 61-year-old patient: one can recognize pale foci between the equator and the ora serrata getting larger toward the periphery and partly surrounded by a delicate pigmented border. The fundus appears rarefied because of the large pale foci. Occasional choroidal vessels are faintly visible. The other eye showed identical changes. The peripheral visual field margins, and the visual acuity were normal on both sides.

**Fig. 144 and 145. Further examples of the dry form of arteriosclerotic chorioretinopathy, large surface type.** Whereas in Fig. 144 one can see in the right eye of a 76-year-old patient large partially confluent, mostly round, depigmented foci with a pigmented border, especially in the central fundus an analogous picture is visible in the outer periphery of the 47-year-old patient in Fig. 145. Experience has taught that the latter changes can lead to retinal hole formation. Arteriosclerosis thus constitutes an important aetiological factor in the development of retinal detachment. Remarkable are the pale lipid deposits within, as well as at the margins of the arteriosclerotic lesions (Fig. 144).

67

**Fig. 146. Onset of the wet-type of arteriosclerotic chorioretinopathy; left eye.** In the wet-form of arterio-sclerotic chorioretinopathy, haemorrhages and oedema occur mainly in the macula region, so that the fundus picture can be quite colourful. In the case presented (fundus of a 55-year-old patient with B.P. 120/70 mm Hg) one can see the onset of the wet stage with only just visible oedema in the central fundus area and delicate almost plaque-like pigmentation. Visual acuity: 5/10.

**Fig. 147 and 148. Varying forms and degrees of arteriosclerotic chorioretinopathy in the right and left eye of the same 49-year-old patient.** In the right eye (Fig. 147) is a slightly prominent pseudo-tumourous cockade-like lesion surrounded by, and interspersed with haemorrhages (the so-called plaque-like degeneration of the central retina of Junius-Kuhnt), as an extreme sign of a sclerotic circulatory disorder. This picture belongs to the wet-form of arteriosclerotic chorioretinopathy. On the left eye (Fig. 148) contrary to this, is a dry arteriosclerotic degeneration with marked small-spotted pigmented and depigmented areas. Vision on the right: finger-counting in 1 m; on the left: 5/5. Sclerotic fundus changes cannot always be exactly divided into one or the other category according to the signs; there is naturally, not infrequently a mixed picture, in which one also finds transitional changes from the dry to the wet forms.

**Fig. 149 and 150. Other examples of the wet-form of arteriosclerotic chorioretinopathy.** The exudative phenomena stand in the foreground in both cases. In the right eye (Fig. 149), the macula is the site of a yellow, sharply demarcated, slightly prominent lesion larger than the optic disc, which contains fine haemorrhages. In the left eye (Fig. 150), is a similarly prominent macula lesion surrounded by, and partially covered with haemorrhages, around which a delicate pigmented halo has formed. Around this area there are also fine radially orientated degenerative lesions, which remind one of a so-called developing circinate retinopathy.

68

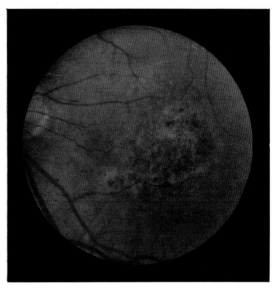

**146**

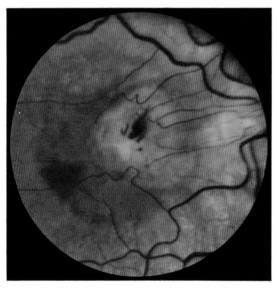

**147**

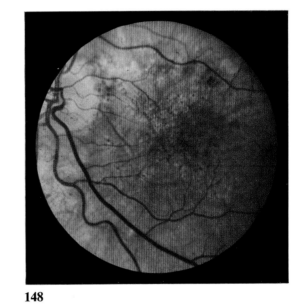

**148**

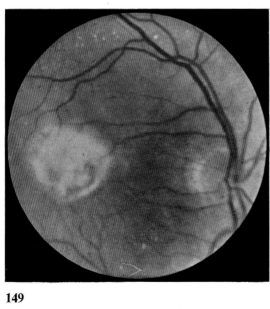

**149**

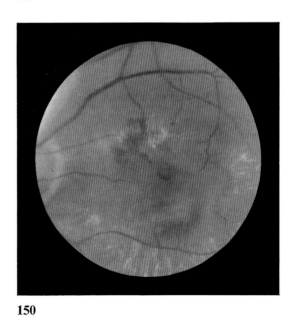

**150**

**Fig. 151–154. Further examples of the wet-type of arteriosclerotic chorioretinopathy.** The colourful signs of this form of arteriosclerosis are presented in these pictures. Pale confluent foci alternate with haemorrhages of varying density and with whitish yellow areas. Especially in later stages, one often sees subretinal concave veil-like fibrinous bands as a sign of proliferative change (Fig. 153 compare also Fig. 164). In these eyes visual acuity was never more than 5/50.

**Fig. 155 and 156. Arteriosclerotic macular degeneration, wet-form; right and left eye of the same 71-year-old patient.** Not infrequently a proliferation characterized by organisation and scarring of connective tissue and glial elements respectively add to the exudation. As is just recognizeable here in the right eye (Fig. 155), these can lead to tumour-like, indistinctly bounded growths. The clinical history showed that the onset of the process in the left eye (Fig. 156) occurred much earlier: the disease began here 2 years previously with a decrease in visual acuity. The central area of the fundus is transformed into an elongated oval, slightly prominent and sharply demarcated scar. The haemorrhage caps the temporal inferior scar margin. Further mostly striped scarred areas lie between the optic disc and the macula. Visual acuity: right 5/20, left 1/35.

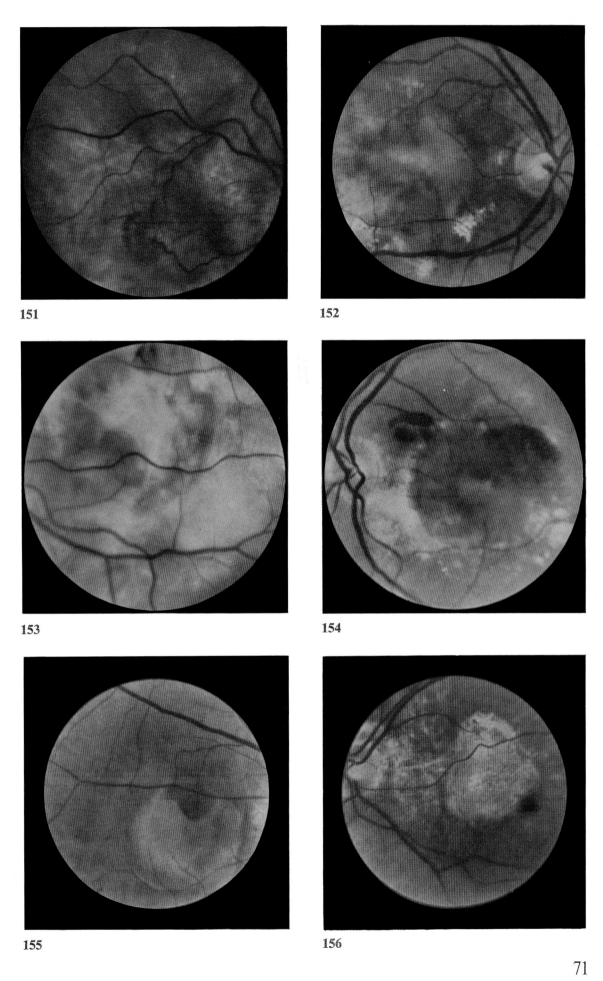

151

152

153

154

155

156

71

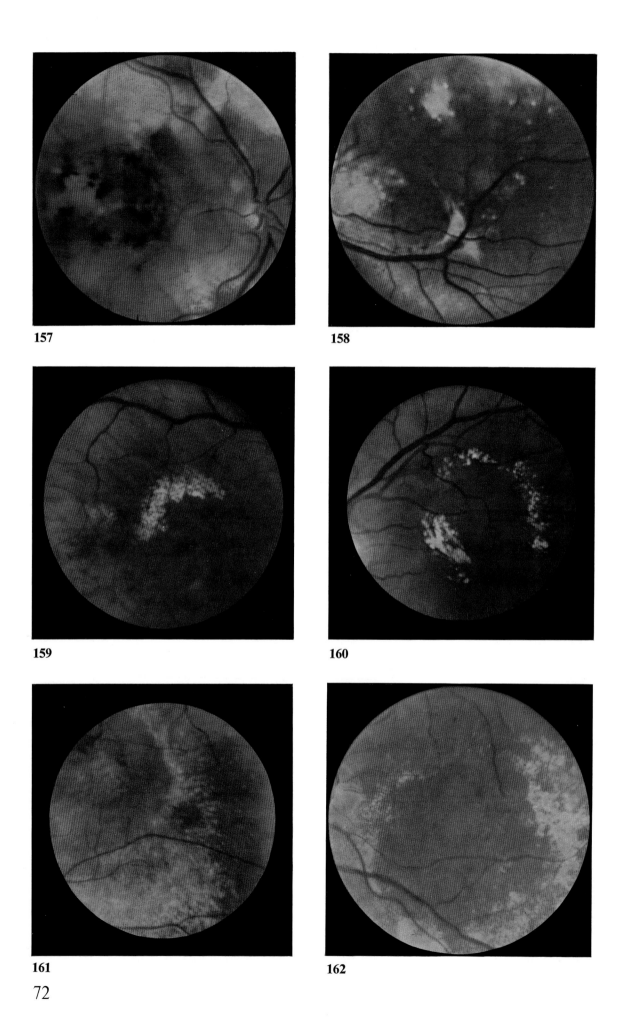

**157**

**158**

**159**

**160**

**161**

**162**

**Fig. 157 and 158. Wet arteriosclerotic fundus changes; right and left eye of the same patient.** This 63-year-old patient complained of decrease in visual acuity for over a year. Visual acuity: right 1/50, left 5/25. On both sides there are severe diffuse sclerotic changes with widespread yellow exudates; on the right eye (Fig. 157), more diffusely cloudy; on the left eye (Fig. 158), slightly more distinct. Also on the right side is an irregular pigmentation in the macula region, and on the left side several fine haemorrhages adjacent to the inferior temporal vascular arc.

**Fig. 159–162. Further cases of arteriosclerotic fundus lesions.** In the wet-form of arteriosclerotic chorioretinopathy, garland-like yellow-white foci can occur which form a more or less complete wreath of varying width around the macula (so-called circinate retinopathy). This just like the plaque-like degeneration of the central retina of Junius-Kuhnt is not obligatory for the diagnosis of arteriosclerotic changes. It is explained on the basis of scarring and organisation of glial and connective tissue elements respectively. In Fig. 161 there is also a marked change of the central retina in the form of fine haemorrhages and hyper- and depigmented zones.

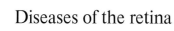

**Fig. 163–165. Proliferative sclerotic fundus changes.** These pictures belong to the wet-form of arterio-sclerotic chorioretinopathy, and show again the manifold appearance of this disease. Circinate retinal changes need not be necessarily confined to the macula region, but can occasionally reach far into the periphery (Fig. 163). In other cases (Fig. 164), one finds sail-like membraneous lesions. In Fig. 165 there are also occasional glittering cholesterol deposits in the centre of several dysoric foci.

**Fig. 166 and 167. So-called plaque-like degeneration of Junius-Kuhnt in the central retina; left eye of a 55-year-old patient with generalized arteriosclerosis.** At first a senile pseudotumour seen in Fig. 166 in the form of a broad, mainly round, pale, prominent area at the posterior pole was seen, which spread over the temporal superior vascular arc. At the inferior margin are delicate remnants of haemorrhages. 9 months later (Fig. 167), the lesion has become more flat and "softer" looking and a subretinal sail-like connective tissue growth has taken its place. The haemorrhage at the lower border has been completely resorbed. Such progress however, must not be regarded as the effect of treatment, as it also occurs spontanously.

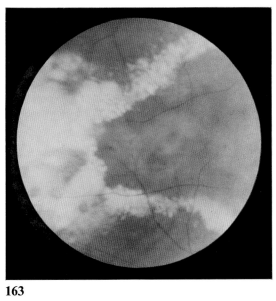

163

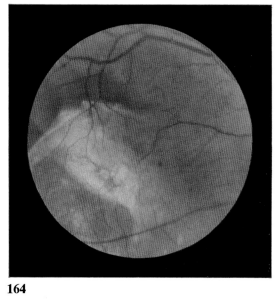

164

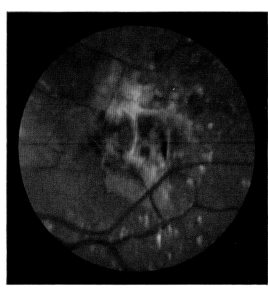

165

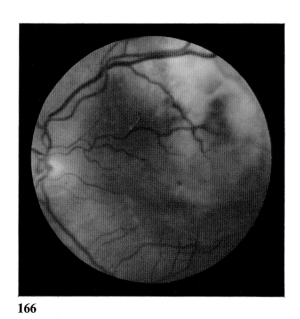

166

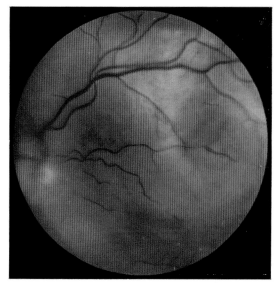

167

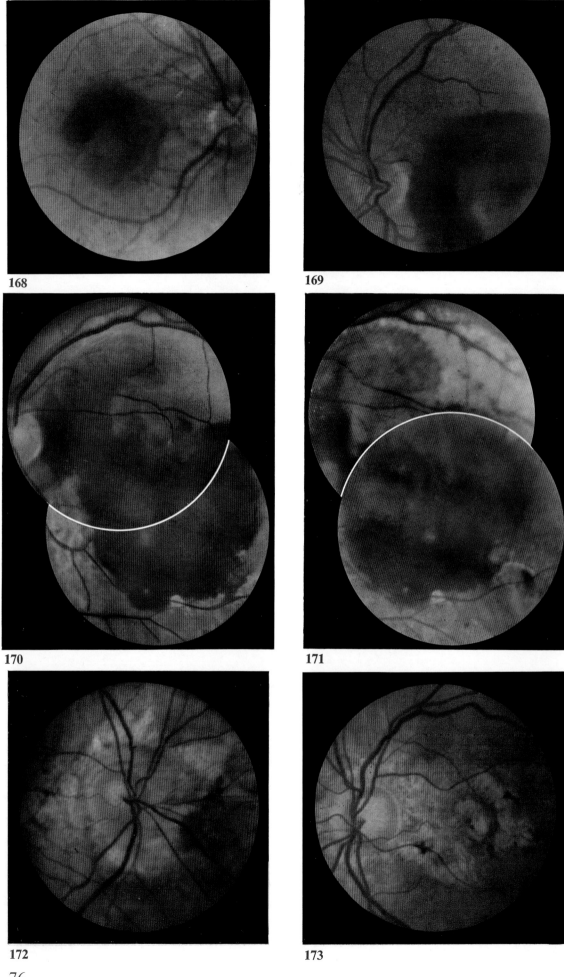

168

169

170

171

172

173

76

**Fig. 168 and 169. Examples of arteriosclerotic macular haemorrhages.** In arteriosclerosis as well, haemorrhages favour the anatomically and functionally especially differentiated area of the posterior pole. They occur in varying size. In some cases one sees small cockade-like forms (Fig. 168), which correspond to the varying density and location of the haemorrhage, and in other cases the haemorrhage reaches the optic disc. In the case shown in Fig. 169 (of a 77-year-old patient with severe general vascular sclerosis), the haemorrhage is mostly preretinal. In the centre the haemorrhage is paler showing the onset of resorption which dates the occurrence of the haemorrhage to quite some time ago.

**Fig. 170 and 171. Arteriosclerotic macular haemorrhage; left eye.** This 55-year-old patient suffered from a sudden decrease in visual acuity on the left eye a month ago. A large mainly preretinal surface haemorrhage of varying density, which covers the retinal vessels, dominates the picture. It hangs almost drop-like under the macula, surrounding the latter with arc-like spurs nasally and superiorly. An increased (sclerotic) tabulation of the choroidal vessels is also visible. At the edge of the haemorrhage there are pale foci in several places. 14 days later (Fig. 171), the haemorrhage although not smaller in size, shows a difference in its colouring as well as a circinate retinopathy at its superior edge.

**Fig. 172 and 173. Arteriosclerotic fundus; right and left eye of the same patient.** A 61-year-old patient with peripapillary choroidal sclerosis on both sides. On the left side there is also an arteriosclerotic macular degeneration with occasional fine haemorrhages and delicate pigmentation in the depigmented area.

77

**Fig. 174. Circumscribed choroidal sclerosis; right eye.** The whole fundus need not always be equally affected. This 72-year-old patient has an almost complete sclerosis of the choroidal vessels in the area around the optic disc as well as in those sections that lie temporally superiorly and inferiorly including the macula. This zone appears remarkably arc-like, and due to its pallor (sclera visible) contrasts with the otherwise normally coloured, tabulated fundus. At the edge of the choroidal sclerosis near the optic disc, one can see choroidal vessels partially filled with blood, with irregular pigment accumulations between them. There is a certain similarity to myopic atrophy; this eye is however emmetropic. This cannot be a case of choroideremia as the electroretinogram was normal. There was an analogous finding on the left side.

**Fig. 175–177. Subretinal arteriosclerotic macular haemorrhage; right eye.** This 71-year-old patient has suffered from cerebral and coronary sclerosis for several years. A decrease in visual acuity occurred on the right to 5/20 20 days ago. In the macula and superior to it there is a wide-spread haemorrhage of typical slate-grey appearance (Fig. 174), with a small oval preretinal haemorrhage at its nasal margin. 4 months later the subretinal haemorrhage has been practically resorbed (Fig. 175). At the previous inferior margin there are now fine yellowish white degenerative areas. Temporal and superior is an arc-like remnant of the haemorrhage with a discrete pigmentary border. Compared to this the preretinal haemorrhage at first shows very little signs of resorption, probably because the retina presents only a relatively small resorptive surface when compared to the choroid. After a further 11½ months (Fig. 176), complete resorption of the haemorrhages. The earlier haemorrhages are now marked by a belt of pigmentation, which reminds one of nevoid retinal pigmentation (compare Fig. 27), but which can be differentiated from the latter by their circular arrangement and the more intense accumulation of pigment which they surround.

**Fig. 178. Choroidal sclerosis is a well-known aspect of general arteriosclerosis.** The choroidal vessels are obliterated, becoming yellow or grey-white. The intervascular spaces (so-called senile tabulation) thus stand out in contrast. The intensity, localisation and size of the changes can vary. In the following cases the choroidal sclerosis is diffuse and encompasses all parts of the fundus.

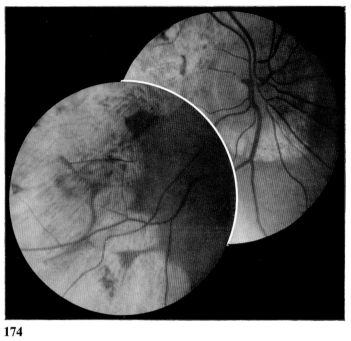

**174**

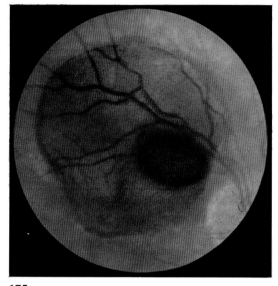

**175**

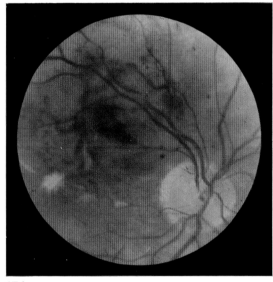

**176**

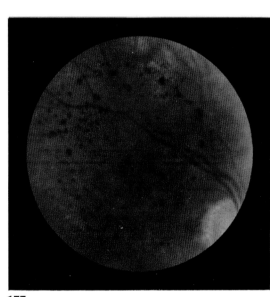

**177**

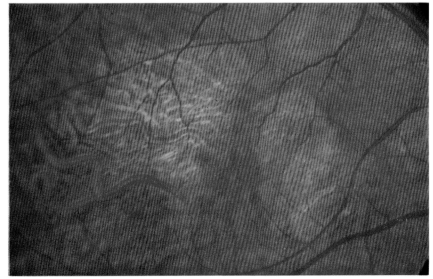

**178**

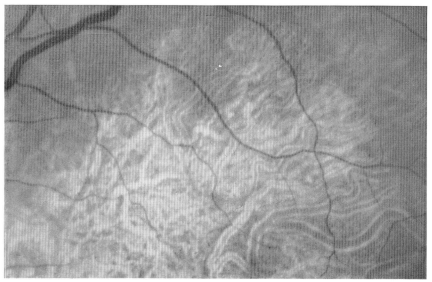

**179**

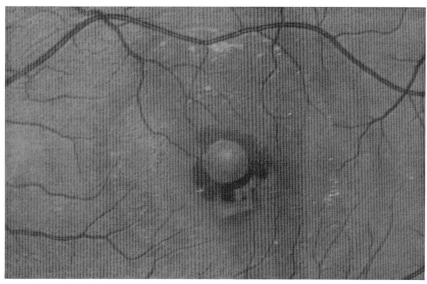

**180**

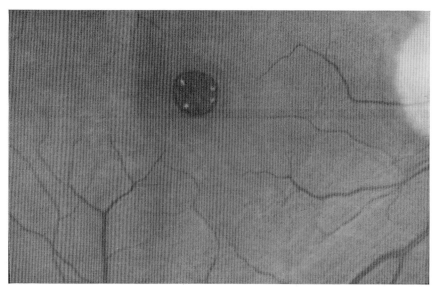

**181**

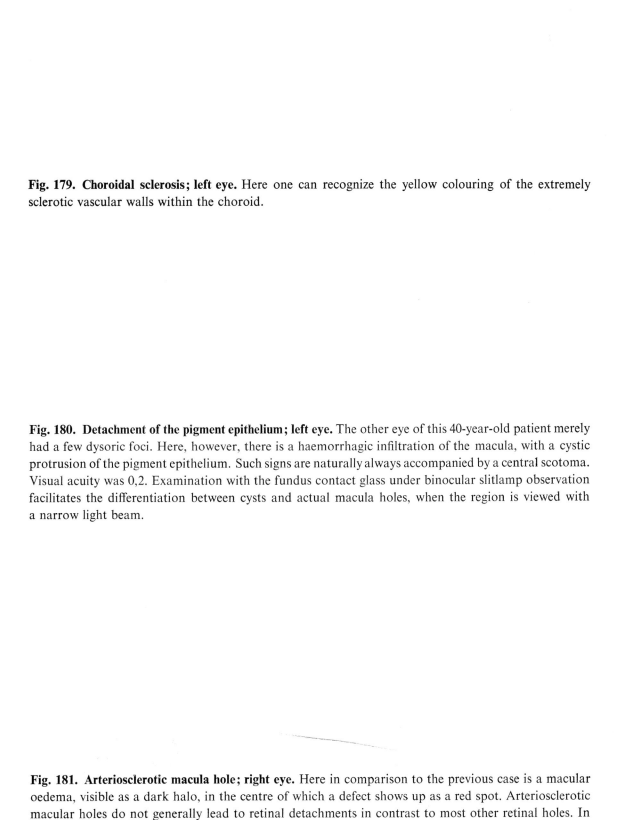

**Fig. 179. Choroidal sclerosis; left eye.** Here one can recognize the yellow colouring of the extremely sclerotic vascular walls within the choroid.

**Fig. 180. Detachment of the pigment epithelium; left eye.** The other eye of this 40-year-old patient merely had a few dysoric foci. Here, however, there is a haemorrhagic infiltration of the macula, with a cystic protrusion of the pigment epithelium. Such signs are naturally always accompanied by a central scotoma. Visual acuity was 0,2. Examination with the fundus contact glass under binocular slitlamp observation facilitates the differentiation between cysts and actual macula holes, when the region is viewed with a narrow light beam.

**Fig. 181. Arteriosclerotic macula hole; right eye.** Here in comparison to the previous case is a macular oedema, visible as a dark halo, in the centre of which a defect shows up as a red spot. Arteriosclerotic macular holes do not generally lead to retinal detachments in contrast to most other retinal holes. In this eye the margins of the macula hole were stabilized by four Argon-laser coagulation foci.

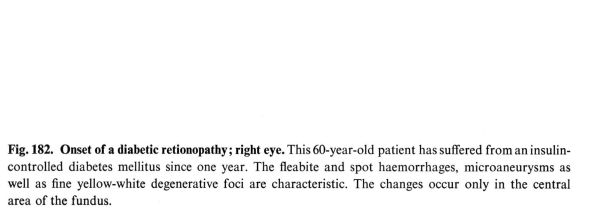

**Fig. 182. Onset of a diabetic retionopathy; right eye.** This 60-year-old patient has suffered from an insulin-controlled diabetes mellitus since one year. The fleabite and spot haemorrhages, microaneurysms as well as fine yellow-white degenerative foci are characteristic. The changes occur only in the central area of the fundus.

**Fig. 183. Diabetic retinopathy, left eye.** Although diabetes was discovered only 3 years ago in this 57-year-old patient one can already see multiple fleabitelike haemorrhages and microaneurysms. They have not as yet led to an objective decrease in visual function.

**Fig. 184. Diabetic retinopathy; right eye of a 69-year-old patient.** Here are the first signs of a diabetic retinopathy: fleabite-like haemorrhages and microaneurysms. In the centre one can recognize the onset of so-called hard exudates. There are often accompanying signs of hypertension and/or arteriosclerosis respectively: varicosity and stasis, as well as irregular calibration of the venules, with broad arterial reflexes.

**Fig. 185. Extreme diabetic retinopathy; right eye.** This patient suffered from diabetes since 20 years. The haemorrhages are in the background, the picture being more one of yellow-white degenerative lesions arranged in a circinate pattern at the posterior pole, which gradually decrease toward the periphery.

**Fig. 186. Onset of proliferative retinopathy; left eye.** As a late sign in diabetic retinopathy, proliferative vitreal strands can occur as here nasal to the optic disc, which ultimately lead to retinal detachment via traction.

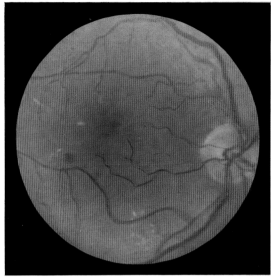

**182**

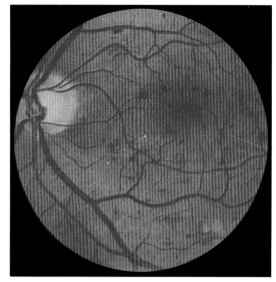

**183**

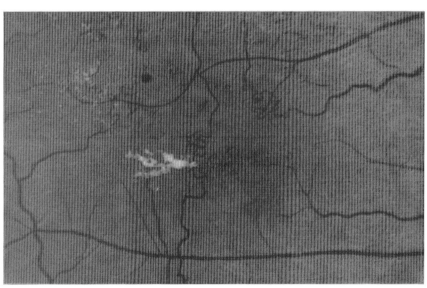

**184**

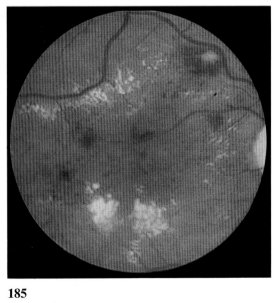

**185**

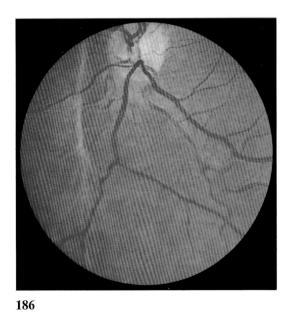

**186**

83

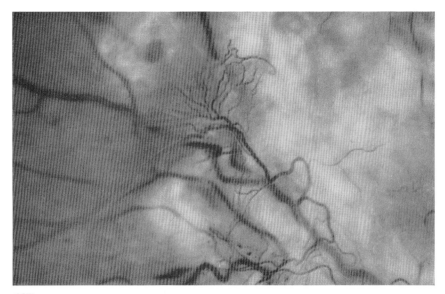

**187**

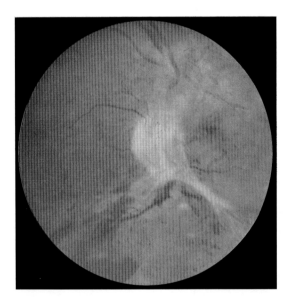

**188**

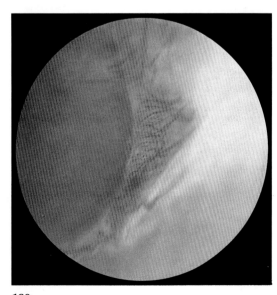

**189**

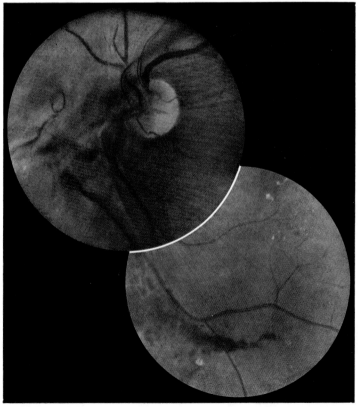

**190**

**Fig. 187. Proliferative diabetic retinopathy in a 35-year-old patient; left eye.** This patient has had diabetes since his 11th year of life. The left eye is now almost completely blind. One can recognize a proliferative vitreal strand arising from the optic disc, and coursing nasally and superiorly, as well as a retinal oedema which partially obliterates the irregular retinal vessels. Dot and stripe haemorrhages are also present.

**Fig. 188. Proliferative diabetic retinopathy; left eye.** Here is a late stage of diabetic retinopathy. There is a triangular sail-like vitreal connective tissue strand arising from the optic disc and surrounded by haemorrhages.

**Fig. 189. Massive proliferative diabetic retinopathy; right eye.** Added to the changes seen in the previous pictures, there are here innumerable newly-formed vessels, which represent a particular danger for the eye: the resulting haemorrhages from these vessels into the vitreous lead to further connective tissue strands which cause a retinal detachment via traction.

**Fig. 190. Severe proliferative diabetic retinopathy; left eye.** This 25-year-old patient has suffered from diabetes mellitus since childhood. At the nasal margin of the optic disc are the beginnings of a proliferative retinopathy with traction of the retinal vessels and stripe like spot haemorrhages. Temporally the retina is still attached. However the onset of a detachment is seen here in the form of fine radial folds. The part of the retina with proliferative changes is sharply demarcated from the attached retinal areas below the optic disc. A partly preretinal, partly intraretinal haemorrhage stretches arc-like from the retinal strands into the temporal part of the fundus, along the inferior temporal vein. As a sign of the circulatory disorder one can just visualize rete mirabile-like vascular anastomosis on the optic disc. 5 months later, there was complete retinal detachment.

**Fig. 191. Fresh periphlebitis; left eye.** This 21-year-old patient came to the eye-clinic because of a corneal foreign body. During examination this abnormal varicosity in the region of a temporal venous retinal branch was found. There are delicate intraretinal spot haemorrhages in the neighbourhood of this area.

**Fig. 192. Periphlebitis; right eye.** In the area of the temporal inferior vein there is circumscribed striped sheathing, and in parts overlay of the venous branch. Earlier on there were radial haemorrhages at this point, which resorbed after treatment in a spa. Other changes were absent.

**Fig. 193. Retinal periphlebitis; right eye.** The diseased fundus areas were treated with Xenon light-coagulation 3 weeks previously. In the area of the still relatively weakly pigmented, but already demarcated light coagulation foci are delicate haemorrhages and new vessel rete mirabile formations.

**Fig. 194. Periphlebitis with posterior uveitis; right eye.** Here there is a broad sheathing of the superior vein, which covers it practically to the equator. Next to this, there are old, sharply demarcated, juxta-papillary retino-choroiditic foci. The simultaneous occurrence of chorioretinitis and periphlebitis indicates a similar aetiology for both diseases.

**Fig. 195. Proliferative retinopathy with periphlebitis and posterior uveitis; right eye.** At the inferior optic disc margin is the onset of a tractional bullous retinal detachment. Formerly there were periphlebitic changes in the periphery. Choroiditic scars are seen nasally and temporally superior to the optic disc. In the region of the superior optic disc margin are delicate stripe haemorrhages.

**Fig. 196. Proliferative retinopathy with periphlebitis; left eye.** The lower half of the retina is mostly affected. There is a corrugated retinal detachment under the optic disc which has occurred through traction of a broad pale scarred strand, which is visible in the left part of the picture. This strand attaches directly to the detached retina with thread-like spurs. The vessels climb over the prominence. In the right inferior part of the picture one sees stripe-like white reflexes at the slope of the retinal detachment nearest to the ora serrata.

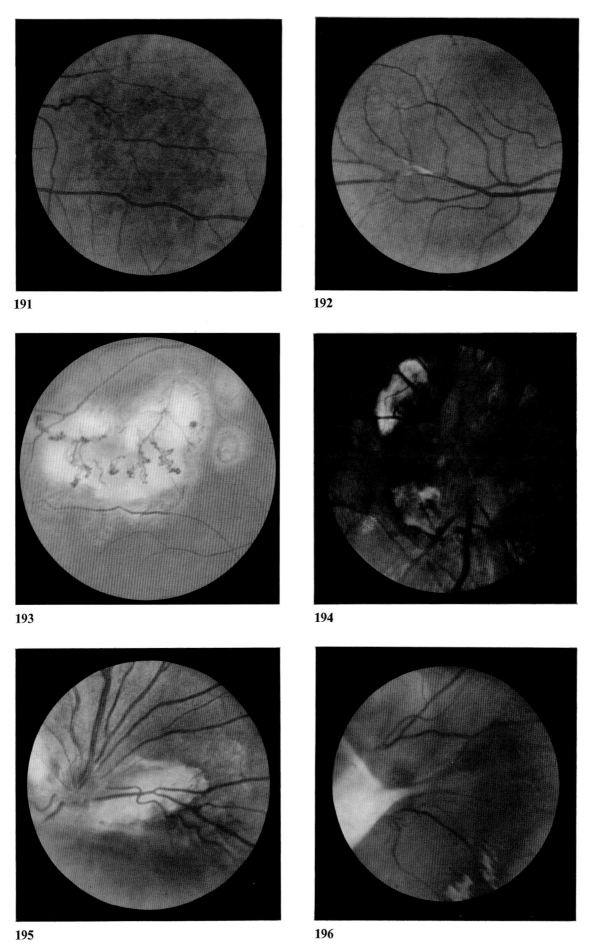

191

192

193

194

195

196

87

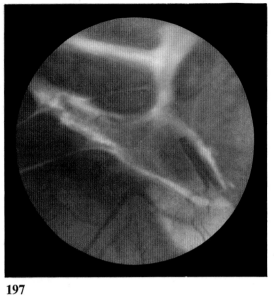

**197**

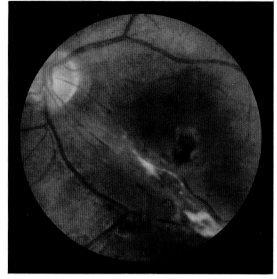

**198**

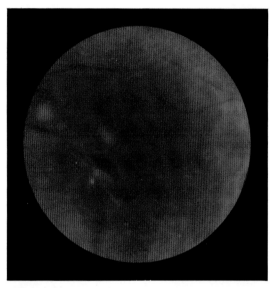

**199**

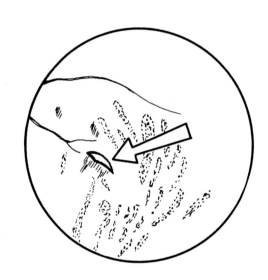

**199 a**

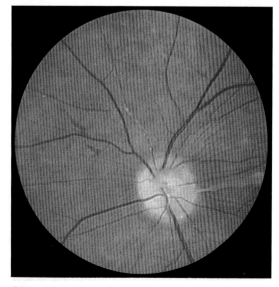

**200**

**Fig. 197. Proliferative retinopathy with periphlebitis; right eye.** Here the superior half of the retina is mainly affected. At the right inferior margin of the picture one can recognize the optic disc from which a vein courses for a short distance in a temporal superior direction, then forming a hairpin-like bend reaches the nasal superior optic disc margin. Other retinal vessels also show an irregular distribution. Net-like broad and narrow strands in the vitreous attach to the optic disc and to the fundus directly above it.

**Fig. 198. Proliferative retinopathy with periphlebitis and a macular hole; left eye.** The periphlebitic changes are located at the temporal inferior vascular arc. Note the circumscribed sheathing and covering of the vessels in this area visible together with the onset of retinal detachment. Haemorrhages which were present earlier, are now resorbed. There is a depigmented focus in the macula with condensation of pigment at its inferior margin. The small macular hole present does not show up in this photograph. Undoubtedly it occurred due to traction of the preretinal scarred tissue strand directly next to it.

**Fig. 199. Peripheral retinal tear with periphlebitis; left eye.** Due to a preretinal connective tissue strand, a small oval retinal hole (sketch) has originated in the terminal area of supply of a small venous branch, in whose neighbourhood delicate white foci are visible. In other areas (not shown here) there are haemorrhages and sheathing of blood vessels.

**Fig. 200. Continuous reversible arteriopathy (Kyrieleis); left eye.** This disease leads to white sheathing of the arterial retinal vascular system. Here the nasal superior artery is involved. An iridocyclitis can also occur. The disease process is reversible, its cause is unknown. An allergic aetiology is suspected.

Inflammatory lesions

**Fig. 201 and 202. Septic retinitis; right and left eye of the same patient.** This 55-year-old patient suffered from a therapy-resistent subacute bacterial endocarditis. 14 days after the onset of the first symptoms, there appeared in the right fundus (Fig. 201), and 4 days later in the left, circumscribed, slightly prominent, indistinct yellow white foci, in close proximity to the retinal vessels. These are in all probability septic metastasis.

**Fig. 203. Fresh juxtapapillary retino-choroiditis of Jensen; left eye.** A sector-shaped visual field defect, or a Bjerrum scotoma corresponding to the localisation of the focus is characteristic for this disease. In the fundus of this 21-year-old patient an indistinct yellowish white round focus with fine haemorrhages at its inferior margin, lies at the temporal edge of the optic disc.

**Fig. 204. Fresh "juxtapapillary" retino-choroiditis of Jensen; left eye in a 28-year-old patient.** An oval indistinct focus lies in the nasal superior periphery. Contrary to opinions expressed until now, such peripheral foci with corresponding visual field defects must be included in the disease entity of Jensen's retinitis. We believe that the diagnosis Jensen's disease is not confined to those foci lying directly at the optic disc. Recent experience has shown that a considerable percentage of all patients in their third decade with focal choroiditis really represent cases of Jensen's retinitis.

**Fig. 205 and 206. Recurrent Jensen retino-choroiditis; right eye of a 37-year-old patient.** This greatly enlarged photograph shows an old sharply demarcated pigmented Jensen focus in the area of supply of a small temporal superior venous branch (Fig. 205). At the superior margin of the lesion is a fresh retinochoroiditis having a yellow colour. 25 days later (Fig. 206), one can see that the oedema has been resorbed, and that there is an onset of pigmentation with a sharp demarcation of the recurrent focus. Perimetry showed that this lesion corresponded to Jensen's disease, even though it resembled the ordinary form of choroiditis.

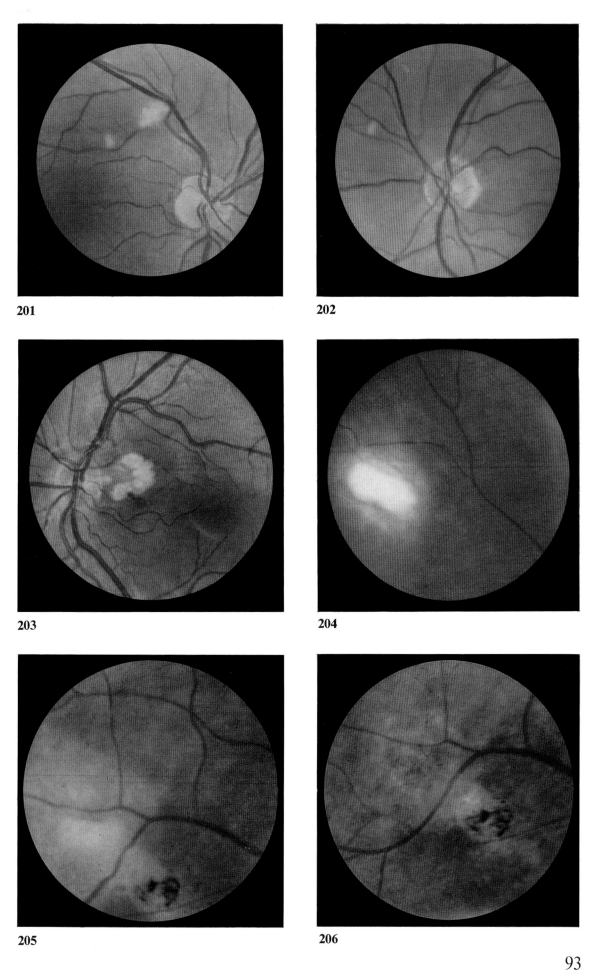

201

202

203

204

205

206

93

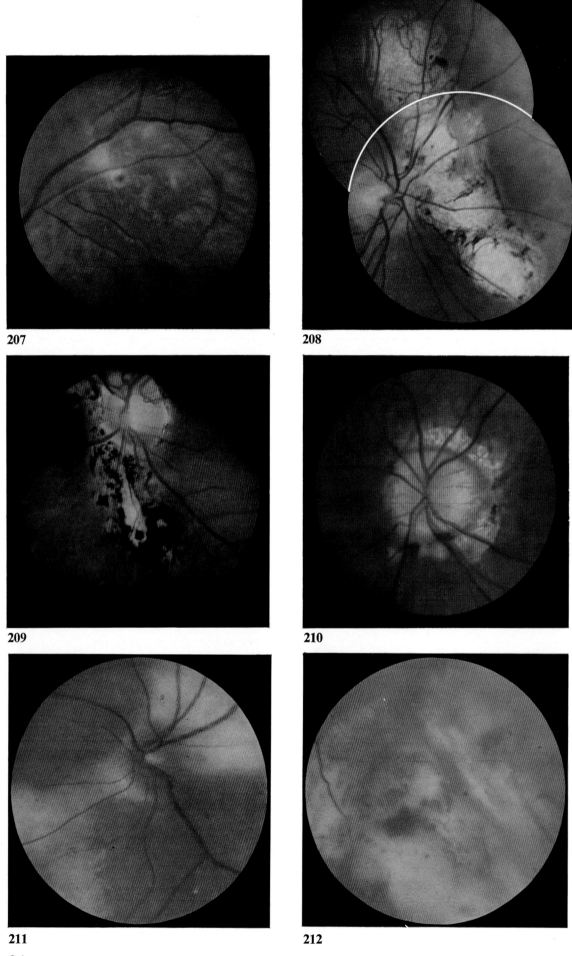

207

208

209

210

211

212

94

**Fig. 207. Recurrent Jensen's retinitis; left eye.** This 15-year-old patient had an old small spotted retino-choroiditic focus in the region of the temporal superior vascular arc. It is visible as a delicate darker circumscribed spot beneath the temporal superior vein. A fresh recurrence has arisen at the superior margin of the lesion. Several further small Jensen foci can be seen temporal to this.

**Fig. 208. Old retino-choroiditis; right eye.** Here a striped scar is in contact with the optic disc nasally, and almost resembles a rupture of the choroid. The inflammation occurred during the childhood of this now 61-year-old patient.

**Fig. 209. Recurrent juxtapapillary retino-choroiditis; left eye.** This 38-year-old patient first suffered a juxtapapillary retino-choroiditis 20 years ago. At that time there was one inferior focus near the optic disc. In the following years 4 recurrences occurred in all around the optic disc. There is now an extreme concentric visual field constriction due to confluence of the several sector-shaped defects. Circumscribed pigmented scars are visible around the optic disc; the inferior one having the greatest diameter.

**Fig. 210. Old juxtapapillary retino-choroiditis; right eye.** At the superior and inferior border of the optic disc are conus-like old choroiditic foci which converge nasally at the 3 o'clock position. There are no fresh changes visible. Practically the whole temporal visual field is defective.

**Fig. 211 and 212. Exudative external retinitis of Coats; left eye.** Widespread onset of subretinal exudates beginning at the optic disc (Fig. 211). The course of the vessels at the temporal superior optic disc margin, shows that the retina is somewhat prominent here. A broad band of exudate coming from the temporal superior periphery, becomes narrower centrally, spares the optic disc, and broadens shelf-like nasally and inferiorly. Fig. 212 shows a section of the nasal inferior periphery: irregular varicosity of the in some parts newly formed retinal vessels, cloudy and spotty haemorrhages of varying intensity in the yellow-coloured zone. The other eye is normal.

Diseases of the retina

**Fig. 213. Exudative external retinitis (Coats); right eye of a 20-year-old girl.** Here one sees an extreme varicosity and stasis of the veins as well as the characteristic subretinal yellowish exudates.

**Fig. 214. Older retinitis of Coats; left eye.** 3½ years ago there was a diffuse external exudative retinitis. The oedema has now disappeared. In the area of the temporal superior vascular arc one can recognize circinate retinopathy-like pale degenerative areas lying under the level of the retinal vessels. Fine radial retinal folds are visible superior to the macula, where there is a round subretinal focus.

**Fig. 215–217. Central serous retinitis; right eye.** This disease consists of a circumscribed oedema in the centre of the fundus. This 34-year-old patient noticed a decrease in visual acuity a few days ago. There is a slight, circularly oval oedema in the macula region with loss of reflexes. The fluorescenceangiography (Fig. 216) shows a leakage at the temporal side of the oedematous island, which remains as a bright indistinct spot a few days after Argon-laser-coagulation (Fig. 217). There was rapid resorption of the retinal oedema. 4 weeks later visual acuity had increased from 0,4 to 1,0.

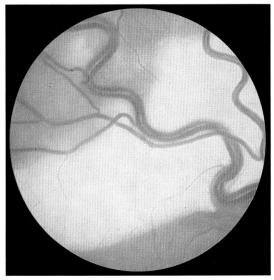

**213**

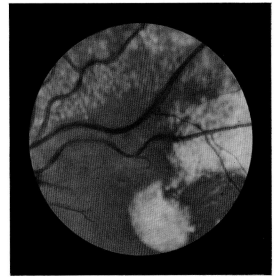

**214**

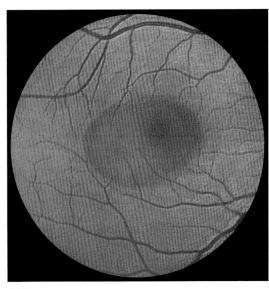

**215**

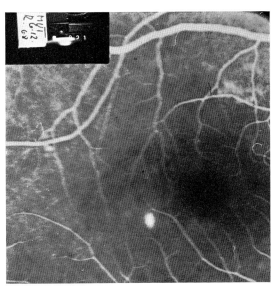

**216**

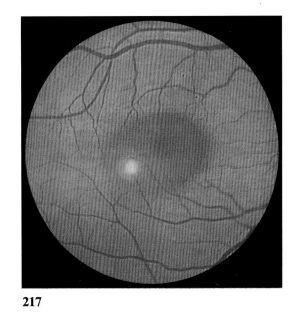

**217**

# Diseases of the haemopoetic system*

\* Strictly speaking Figures 218–221 do not belong to this chapter. However, the fundus changes justify their inclusion in this context.

99

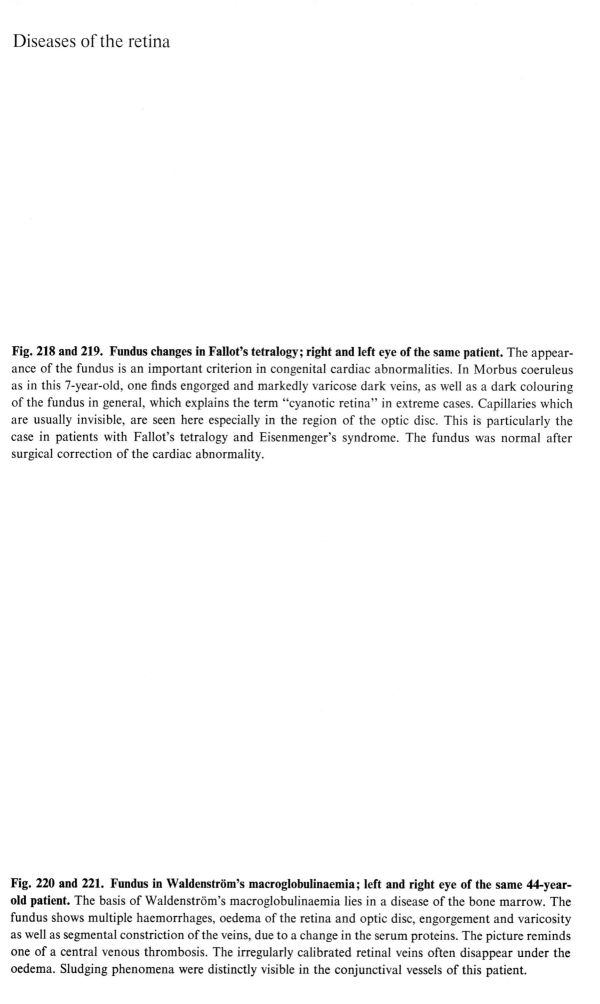

**Fig. 218 and 219. Fundus changes in Fallot's tetralogy; right and left eye of the same patient.** The appearance of the fundus is an important criterion in congenital cardiac abnormalities. In Morbus coeruleus as in this 7-year-old, one finds engorged and markedly varicose dark veins, as well as a dark colouring of the fundus in general, which explains the term "cyanotic retina" in extreme cases. Capillaries which are usually invisible, are seen here especially in the region of the optic disc. This is particularly the case in patients with Fallot's tetralogy and Eisenmenger's syndrome. The fundus was normal after surgical correction of the cardiac abnormality.

**Fig. 220 and 221. Fundus in Waldenström's macroglobulinaemia; left and right eye of the same 44-year-old patient.** The basis of Waldenström's macroglobulinaemia lies in a disease of the bone marrow. The fundus shows multiple haemorrhages, oedema of the retina and optic disc, engorgement and varicosity as well as segmental constriction of the veins, due to a change in the serum proteins. The picture reminds one of a central venous thrombosis. The irregularly calibrated retinal veins often disappear under the oedema. Sludging phenomena were distinctly visible in the conjunctival vessels of this patient.

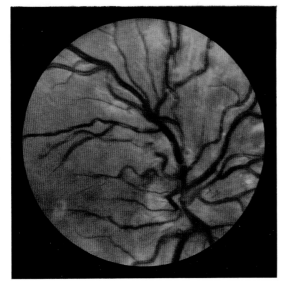

218

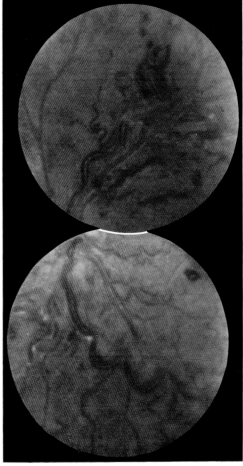

220

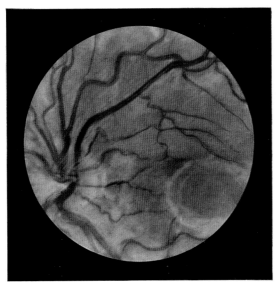

219

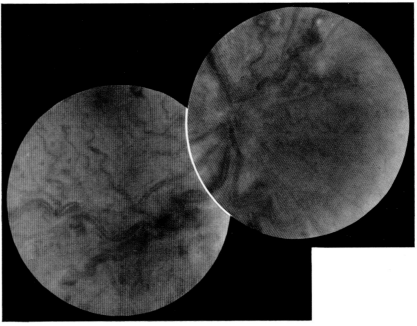

221

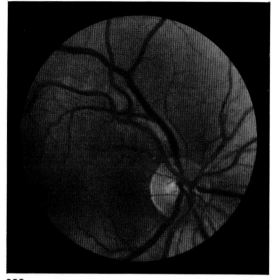

**222**

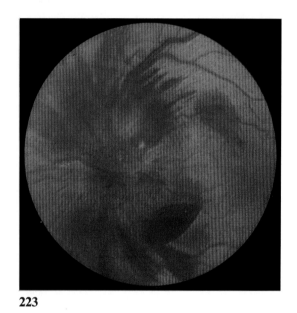

**223**

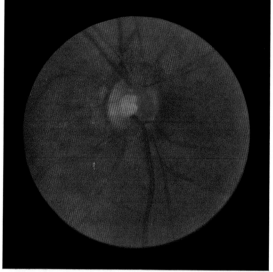

**224**

**225**

**Fig. 222. Polycythaemia rubra vera.** Right eye of a 42-year-old female patient. There is less venous stasis and varicosity in true polycythaemia than in that associated with the venous stasis of emphysema or cardiac abnormalities, where retinal oedema and haemorrhages are also seen. In this case, a genuine polycythaemia rubra vera was found. There is dark coloration of the fundus with some varicosity congestion, and dilatation of the very dark retinal veins. Investigations for polycythaemia should be undertaken in all cases of central retinal vein occlusion.

**Fig. 223. Fundus in haemophilia; left eye.** Diseases of the haemopoetic system can sometimes involve the fundus. Usually there are however no characteristic signs, so that the fundus picture is no aid in the diagnosis of the basic disease process in every case. This case shows massive haemorrhages in the region of the optic disc and the neighbouring retina, especially at the level of the nerve fibre layer. The occasional preretinal haemorrhages can be recognized by their blood levels.

**Fig. 224. Lipaemia retinalis; right eye.** This 50-year-old patient suffers from hypercholesterinaemia, with a total serum cholesterol reaching values up to 943 mg%. Added to this is an increase in serum lipids. Repeated examinations showed extremely pale arteries with broad reflexes as in the picture here.

**Fig. 225. Fundus haemorrhages in cachexia; right eye.** This 74-year-old patient was extremely cachectic with a body weight of 43 kg. Blood pressure was 170/90 mm Hg. The reason was malignant reticuloses. In the foreground are radial striped haemorrhages and a remarkable pallor of the retinal arteries. An engorgement and increased varicosity of the retinal veins is a sign of the sclerotic-hypertensive circulatory disorder also present.

**Fig. 226–228. Fundus changes in lymphogranulomatosis; right and left eye of the same 20-year-old patient.** Note the widespread preretinal haemorrhages which cover the retinal vessels on both eyes. On the left (Fig. 227), one also recognizes somewhat smaller haemorrhages in several places, especially in the region of the macula and directly above it. There is a slightly increased varicosity of some venous branches. Fig. 228 shows how quickly such a picture can change: this is a photograph of the right fundus taken one month after the first. The large surface haemorrhages in the area of the temporal superior artery and the nasal superior artery, as well as another haemorrhage in the 3 o'clock position more peripherally have all become smaller.

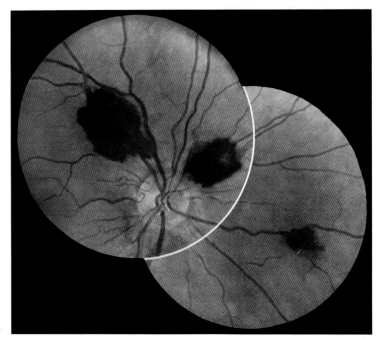

226

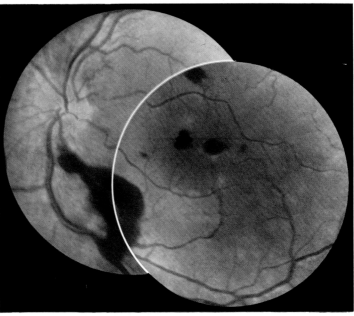

227

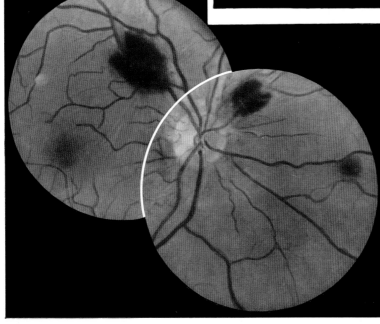

228

Degenerative lesions

**Fig. 229. Retinitis pigmentosa; right eye.** Advanced stage of the disease in a 61-year-old patient. The fine spidery pigmentations resembling bone-corpuscles have encroached towards the centre, and have almost reached the optic disc. The latter is of a waxy pallor and somewhat indistinct. Extreme attenuation of the arterial branches with apparent obliteration of the nasal superior and nasal inferior branches.

**Fig. 230. Disseminated tapeto-retinal degeneration of pigmentosa type; right eye.** Pigmentary changes in this disease are not always of the typical bone-corpuscle configuration. In this case (25-year-old woman), although the clinical course of the disease was similar the pigment is more clumped, analogous changes were found in the other eye.

**Fig. 231 and 232. Disseminated tapeto-retinal degeneration of pigmentosa type; right and left eye of the same patient.** Advanced attenuation of the vessels, which can best be seen by comparing the calibration of the retinal arterial and venous branches with the diameter of the optic disc. Massive choroidal sclerosis with almost complete disappearance of the choroid in places. Bloodfilled choroidal vessels are only present in a few areas especially in the central fundus. Bone-corpuscle-like pigmentation is also absent in the periphery. The disease however corresponds in its course and in loss of function to a pigment degeneration.

**Fig. 233 and 234. Retinitis pigmentosa; right and left eye of the same 19-year-old patient.** Typical waxy yellow optic atrophy with moderate constriction of the vessels. Occasional pigment foci and delicate dot-like pale areas lie in the vicinity of the optic disc. On the right side (Fig. 233), the pigmentation is particularly aggregated along a temporal inferior vessel. Whereas the rest of the central fundus upto the equator is practically absent of all types of pigmentation (these occuring only in the periphery), a widespread atrophy of the choroidal vessels is present as is often the case in this disease. The vessels are visible as bloodless pale lines. There is increased pigmentation of the intervascular choroidal spaces.

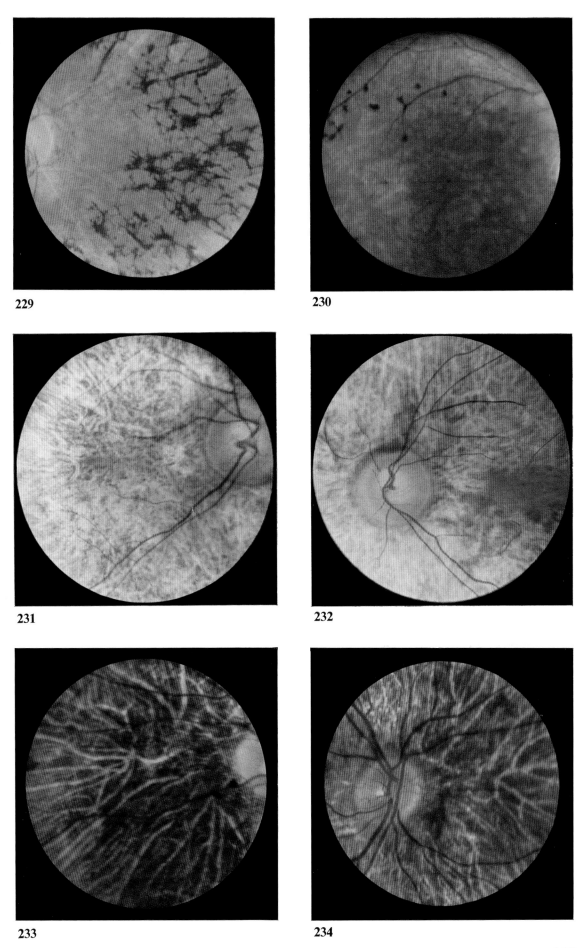

229

230

231

232

233

234

109

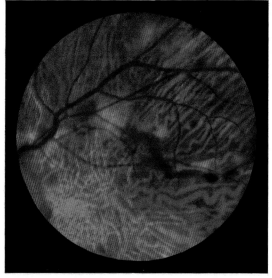

235

Fig. 235. Disseminated tapeto-retinal degeneration of pigmentosa type; left eye. In this patient the pigment is arranged mostly in bands and stripes. Only far out in the periphery are occasional bone-corpuscle-like pigment aggregations. Extreme sclerosis of the choroid especially in the region between the optic disc and the macula. Onset of waxy yellow atrophy of the optic disc with marked constriction of the arterial vascular branches.

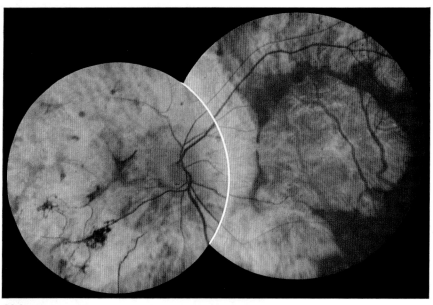

236

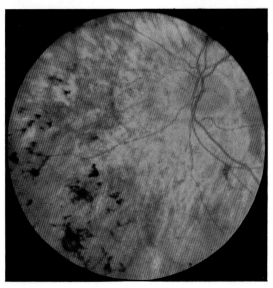

237

Fig. 236 and 237. Retinitis pigmentosa with pathologic myopia; right and left eye of the same 56-year-old patient. Retinitis pigmentosa is often combined with pathologic myopia. – Here extreme disappearance of the choroid at the posterior pole especially on the right side (Fig. 236). The atrophic arc-like zones are partially separated from the rest of the red fundus periphery. There is a more linear choroidal atrophy on the left side (Fig. 237). Bone-corpuscle-like, and delicate branching filigree pigmentation spreads nasally almost to the optic disc.

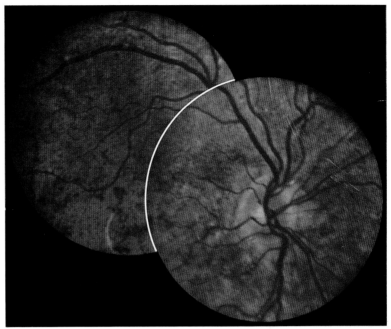

238

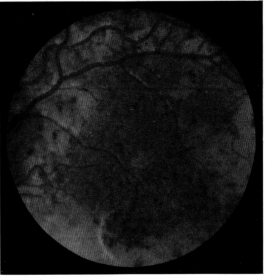

239

**Fig. 238 and 239. Retinitis pigmentosa without pigment; right and left eye of the same 7-year-old patient.**
On both sides there is a ring scotoma and a decrease in intensity and time of the dark-adaptation curve. The electroretinogram is obliterated. There are pepper- and salt-like pigment clumps partially disseminated, partially in groups across the whole fundus, with sparing of the reflexless fovea. There is as yet no recognizable attenuation of the vessels. In some of these cases the typical bone-corpuscle-like pigmentation develops later. Electroretinogram investigations have shown the existence of an ophthalmoscopically identical picture to this disseminated tapeto-retinal degeneration, but with preservation of the retinal potentials and without progressional changes.

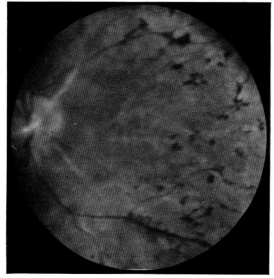

**240**

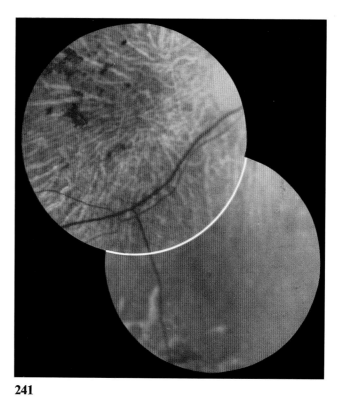

**241**

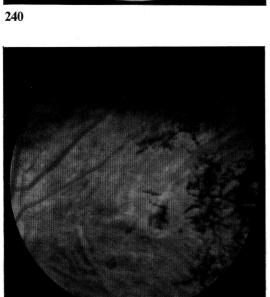

**242**

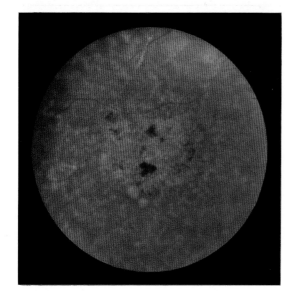

**243**

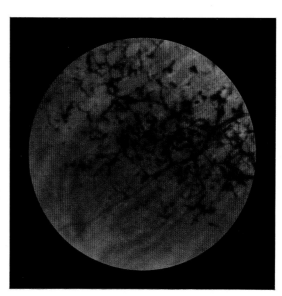

**244**

**Fig. 240. Retinitis pigmentosa with signs of a posterior uveitis; right eye.** A 33-year-old patient with retinitis pigmentosa. Nasally to the optic disc several bone-corpuscle-like pigmentations, which are partially adjacent to the vessels. There are also pale concomitant lines at the entrance of the veins and exit of the arteries respectively, as well as white deposits. These pale concomitant lines are also present occasionally in the periphery. This picture corresponds to a retinal perivasculitis. The preretinal opacities of the vitreous are a further proof of previous inflammation. An analogous picture was found in the other eye. Recent experience leads to the assumption that disseminated tapeto-retinal degenerations of the pigmentosa type can be accompanied by inflammatory changes in the fundus, a fact which seems remarkable when one considers the condition of the retinal and choroidal blood vessels in these degenerative diseases (compare also Fig. 241).

**Fig. 241. Pigment degeneration and simultaneous inflammatory fundus changes; right eye.** Like her mother this patient had a bilateral disseminated tapeto-retinal degeneration of pigmentosa type. The distribution of pigment is somewhat sparse and coarse in this case. There are also old choroiditic foci in the periphery of both eyes. Furthermore as seen in the lower part of the picture, yellow branching inter-anastomosing lines are present. They remind one of a former widespread exudate, somewhat like an external exudative retinitis.

**Fig. 242. Pseudoretinitis pigmentosa; right eye.** Retinitis pigmentosa-like fundus pigmentation can occur after occlusion of the retinal vessels after measles, scarlet fever and various intoxications, as well as congenitally, when the mother has suffered German measles in the first months of pregnancy. This "pseudoretinitis pigmentosa" is not a progressive degeneration, but occurs within a short period of time usually on the basis of a more or less acute localized circulatory disorder, and reaching its final stage after a relatively quick development. Strictly speaking pseudoretinitis pigmentosa does not belong to the chapter of degenerative diseases. The electroretinogram makes the differentiation between a true and a pseudoretinitis pigmentosa possible. Generally in disseminated tapeto-retinal degenerations of pigmentosa type the potentials are extinguished; whereas, they are more or less well preserved in a pseudoretinitis pigmentosa. The aetiology of the disease in the present case was unknown. There are fine bone-corpuscle-like and filigree-like pigmentations, as well as massive clumps of pigment in the whole fundus periphery. Slight attenuation of the vessels is present. The optic disc is unaltered.

**Fig. 243. Central fundus in pseudoretinitis pigmentosa; right eye.** This 41-year-old patient had bone-corpuscle-like pigmentation as well as delicate pale foci in the periphery. The macula is the site of diffuse depigmentation and localized pigment clumping as well as fine yellow confluent foci in its neighbourhood.

**Fig. 244. Pseudoretinitis pigmentosa; right eye.** This picture shows the temporal inferior section of the periphery with fine branching pigmentations partially adjacent to the vessels. An identical picture was found in the other eye. The tests for visual function and the course of the disease showed that this was not a true retinitis pigmentosa. The aetiology is unknown.

**Fig. 245 and 246. Peculiar familial fundus changes; right and left eye of the same patient.** A pale conus-like zone stretches from the right optic disc nasally to the middle periphery and is irregularly demarcated from the rest of the normal coloured fundus periphery (Fig. 245). In this area are pale and grey dots. In the periphery occasional star-shaped pigment deposits; on the left (Fig. 246) there is also a peri-papillary conus-like choroidal atrophy with somewhat attenuated vessels. Visual acuity: right and left eye, 15,0 5/15. The electroretinogram was intact. The mother of this 22-year-old had a typical retinitis pigmentosa, and her two brothers showed similar changes as seen here.

**Fig. 247. Gyrate retinal and choroidal atrophy; right eye.** The differential diagnosis between pathologic myopia and those cases of gyrate atrophy combined with high myopia cannot always be made clinically. Here is a bilaterally identical fundus picture in a 79-year-old patient. The whole fundus is pale. Some choroidal vascular remnants are seen only in the region of the macula and in some areas of the periphery. The retinal vessels course over the spotted pale fundus, and the few intact choroidal vessels are mostly sclerosed. Irregular pigmentations show the dissolution of the retinal pigment epithelium. The optic disc is yellowish.

**Fig. 248. Gyrate atrophy; right eye.** Note the large surface-like disappearance of the choroidal tissue with a few intact islands. The concomitant pathologic myopia is recognizable by the posterior staphyloma-like ectasia of the peripapillary region. The heredity of gyrate atrophy can be dominant or sex-linked recessive.

**Fig. 249. Gyrate atrophy; left eye.** Here the choroid is somewhat more intact when compared to the two previous pictures. On the whole there is however also a widespread disappearance of the choroidal tissue, with obliteration of most of the choroidal vessels. Only some choroidal vessels are filled with blood.

**Fig. 250. Choroideremia; right eye.** This is a disease which is characterized by a progressive disappearance of the choroid beginning in the periphery of the fundus. Only males are affected. The disease begins in youth. At first the macula region and the neighbourhood of the optic disc are spared. Later atrophic islands which slowly become confluent occur in the central areas. The picture can now look very similar to a gyrate atrophy. Anatomical and pathological studies have shown that only the retinal pigment epithelium and the rods and cones with their nuclei are involved in choroideremia. Due to the extinguished retinal potentials in the electroretinogram, choroideremia must be included in the disseminated tapeto-retinal degenerations of pigmentosa type; whereas, gyrate atrophy does not necessarily belong to this group. Here there is a disappearance of choroidal tissue from the optic disc to the periphery. This is a late stage in the disease. Extreme attenuation of the vessels, retinal (ascending) waxy yellow atrophy of the optic disc with slight blurring of its margins. Analogous findings in the other eye as well as in the fundi of this 50-year-old patient's 4-year-younger brother.

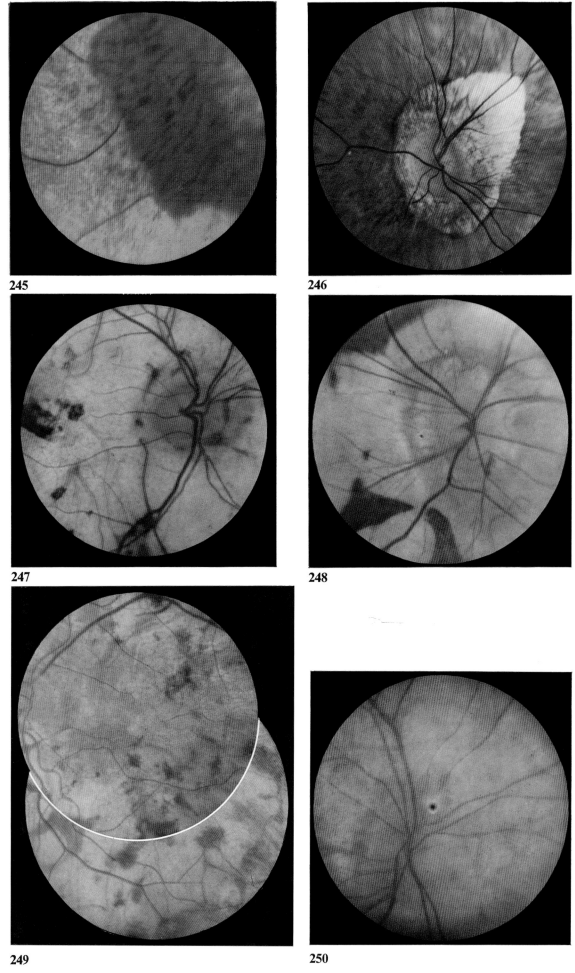

245

246

247

248

249

250

115

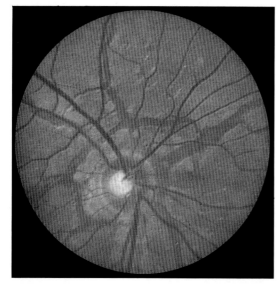

**251**

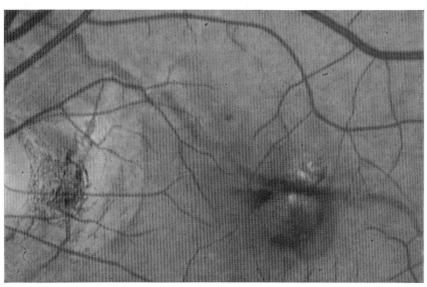

**252**

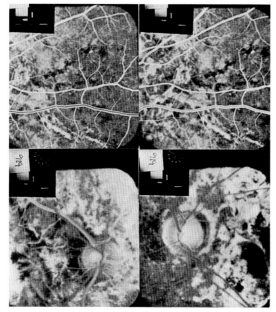

**252 a**

**Fig. 251 and 252. Angioid streaks; right and left eye of the same 28-year-old patient.** Here there are brown stripes lying under the retina, resembling vessels. They are situated more or less concentrically around the optic disc, and from here they run radially into the periphery. The morphological substrate for these changes are tears in Bruch's membrane. In the present advanced case one also sees depigmentary changes in the central retina, as well as pigment clumping and yellow foci forming a pseudotumour under the macula. The pigmentations are partly remnants of previous haemorrhages. This progressive fundus change is most frequently found in combination with pseudoxanthoma elasticum and is a sign of the systemic disease of elastic tissue called Grönblad-Strandberg's syndrome. The fluorescenceangiography (Fig. 252a) shows the angioid streaks as dark stripes.

**Fig. 253. Amaurotic Idiocy; right eye.** Typical fundus in a 1-year-old patient. Cherry-red spot in the fovea surrounded by an oedematous halo. Ascending optic atrophy is a concomitant finding of the severe cerebro-spinal disorder beginning in the first year of life. The aetiology of this disease does not lie within the optic nerve but rather in the retina, where the ganglion cells are destroyed. Blindness results eventually. The disease is fatal in the second or third year of life, due to the increasing loss of ganglion cells within the cerebral tissue. This is a familial disease which especially favours members of the jewish races. A similar form (Stock-Spielmeyer) occurs in children between the 4th and 15th year of life (juvenile amaurotic idiocy).

**Fig. 254. Juvenile macular degeneration; right eye of a 23-year-old patient.** Dark colouring of the central fundus with absent reflexes. In the centre of the retina light areas of a shagreen pattern. Glittering reflexes in the region of the temporal superor vessels.

**Fig. 255 and 256. Juvenile macular degeneration; right and left eye of the same 30-year-old patient.** There is an absence of reflexes in the central fundus where there are cloudy pigmentary changes interspersed with partially confluent paler areas. Visual acuity on both sides: 5/10. The patient had poor visual acuity since childhood.

**Fig. 257 and 258. Juvenile macular degeneration; right and left eye of the same 10-year-old patient.** A youthful fundus rich in reflexes with delicate depigmentary and pigmentary changes in the central area. This results in a cockade-like appearance of the central retina. On the left (Fig. 258) one almost has the impression of a "cherry-red spot" (compare Fig. 253). Findings in both eyes were not quite symmetrical.

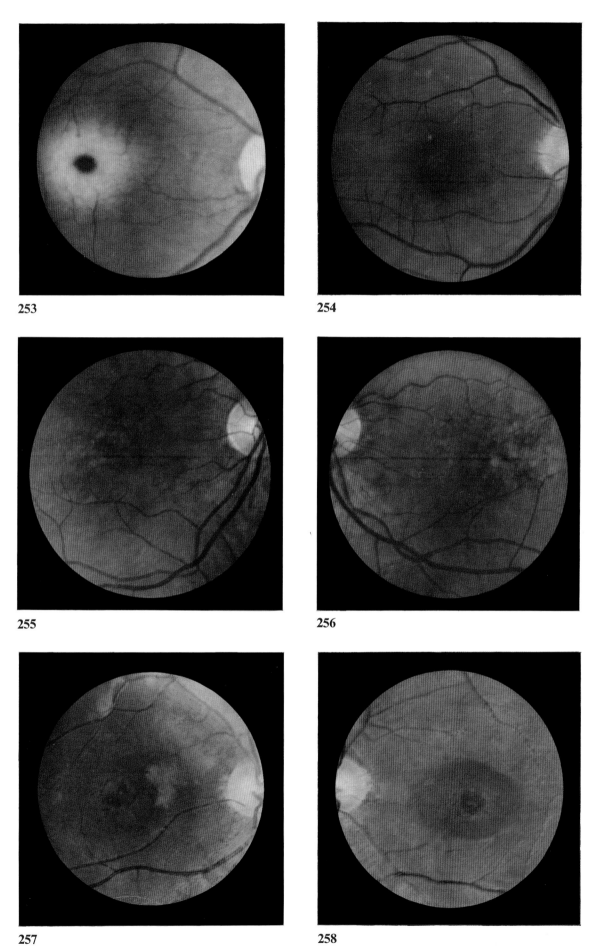

253

254

255

256

257

258

119

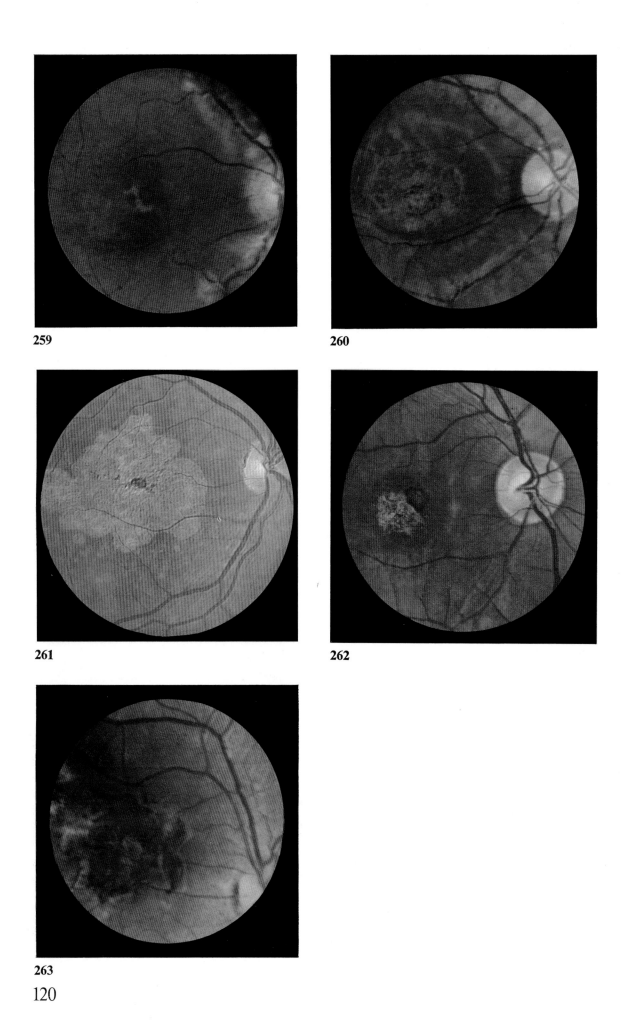

**259**

**260**

**261**

**262**

**263**

120

**Fig. 259–263. Further examples of juvenile macula degeneration.** The manifold appearance of this disease is demonstrated by the following photographs. Whereas Fig. 259 shows a delicate central depigmentation with a fine dark border, the next pictures represent more intense change. In Fig. 260 one can recognize a somewhat more widespread, more marked depigmentary structural change. Fig. 261 shows a surface-like oval sharply demarcated degenerated lesion. Here the choroidal vessels are plainly visible. Irregular pigmentation is also present in the fovea. In Fig. 262 one can see an intense irregular depigmentation of the macula which is sharply demarcated. Pigment lost here has accumulated cap-like at the nasal superior border of this lesion. In comparison to the previous pictures the changes shown in Fig. 263 (of an 11-year-old child) are so marked, that they remind one of a past choroiditis: coarse surface band and clump-like pigment accumulations which are irregularly arranged over the whole macular area and beyond. Certain macular degenerations can develop into disseminated tapeto-retinal degenerations of pigmentosa type. Loss of the b-wave in electroretinogram studies can determine these forms prognostically.

# Retinal detachment

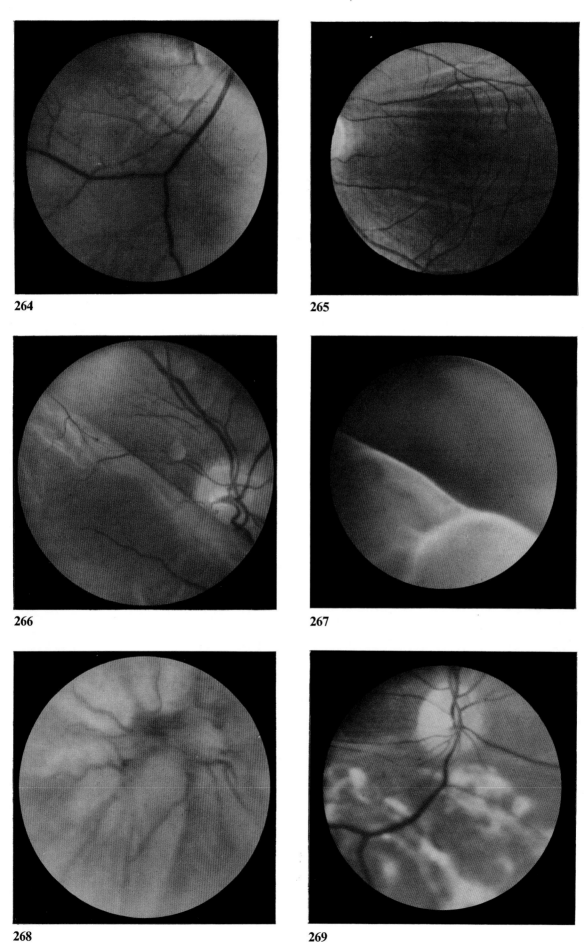

264

265

266

267

268

269

124

**Fig. 264. Onset of retinal detachment; right eye.** Temporally inferior from the optic disc is a so-called pellucid retinal detachment. The retina is only slightly detached and lies in fine folds. Thus the fundus still retains its reddish colouring in this area. Otherwise there is increased darker coloration of the inferior temporal vein.

**Fig. 265. Folding of the retina due to a retrobulbar tumour; left eye.** Here there are almost radially arranged folds running from the optic disc temporally across the central fundus. The cause was an optic nerve sheath meningioma in this 40-year-old patient, which lying within the muscle cone indented the eyeball from behind. Visual acuity: 5/15.

**Fig. 266. Traumatic retinal detachment; right eye.** This patient suffered a contusion of his eyeball $3\frac{1}{2}$ months ago. There is now a detached retina lying in folds in the inferior half, beginning in the temporal superior fundus and proceeding tangentially to the optic disc. The macula is included in the detachment. The detached retina is of a lighter colour compared to the surrounding attached parts. The difference in levels is made visible by the tortuous course of the corresponding vessels.

**Fig. 267. Retinal detachment; left eye.** This 7-year-old girl suffered a retinal detachment without apparent cause in an emmetropic eye. One sees the typical yellowish grey colouring of the prominently detached retinal segments. The attached reddish retina appearing in a different plane is indistinct in this picture.

**Fig. 268. Total retinal detachment; left eye.** Here is a total retinal detachment present since 6 months, after 2 surgical attempts at reattachment. The whole retina is detached in balloon-like waves with a corresponding arrangement of the vessels and a funnel-shaped inversion in the area of the optic disc. After an encircling procedure (after Arruga) the retina was attached. Visual acuity at the time of discharge: 1/35.

**Fig. 269. Old retinal detachment with secondary changes; right eye.** Flat detachment of the inferior half of the retina. This detachment was present since 5 years (!). A considerable part has undergone spontaneous reattachment. There are greyish white cloudy and veil-like degenerative foci partially in, but mostly under the level of the retinal vessels.

**Fig. 270 and 271. Secondary retinal detachment after periphlebitis; right eye.** The nasal part of the fundus (Fig. 270) is indistinct in this picture due to the preretinal vitreal strands and the onset of a retinal detachment. Just nasally from the optic disc there is a greyish connective tissue strand adherent to the retinal surface and following a vertical course. Fig. 271 shows this preretinal vitreal tissue mass in detail. It consists of wing-like sails with window-like "dehiscences" (compare also Fig. 196 and 197).

**Fig. 272. Retinal hole; left eye.** After cataract extraction in this 68-year-old patient, optic phenomena such as flashes of light and mouches volantes were noted. An oval retinal hole was found in the middle periphery. This picture shows the condition a short while after Xenon-light-coagulation.

**Fig. 273. Retinal hole; right eye.** 15 years ago this patient suffered a retinal detachment treated by surgery. The control examination now showed a new horseshoe tear in another area. 5 days ago this was treated with Xenon-coagulation.

**Fig. 274. Condition after encircling procedure (Arruga); right eye.** Prognostically this was a very unfavourable retinal detachment in an 11-year-old patient which was treated surgically 4 times in the past without success. Now a cerclage was performed. The indentation of the sclera is seen as a pigmented wall through which the thread shimmers slightly. The latter was therefore cut through.

**Fig. 275. Condition after prophylactic light coagulation; right eye.** A horseshoe-shaped tear in an attached retina was discovered in the nasal superior periphery as a chance finding on ophthalmoscopy. This picture shows the findings 12 days after surgery. One can just discern the contour of the tear as well as the darker coloured flap. The neighbourhood of the defect is surrounded by light coagulation areas which have almost become scarred. There is a moderate oedema with indistinct margins at the inferior and temporal inferior edges of the tear. This disappeared later.

126

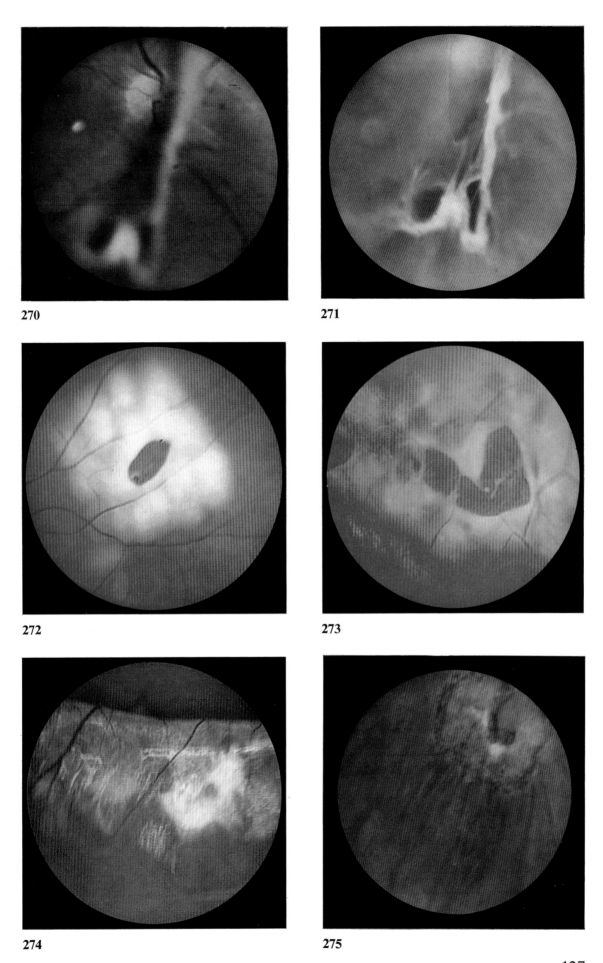

270

271

272

273

274

275

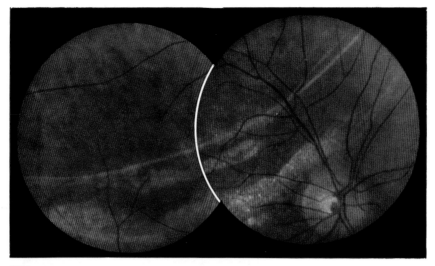

**276**

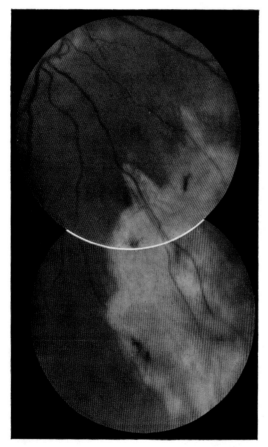

**277**

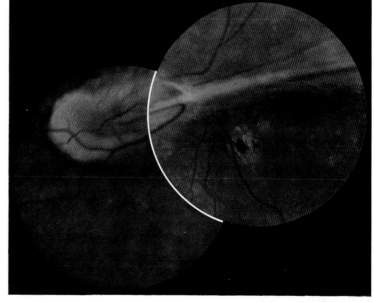

**278**

**Fig. 276. Condition after retinal detachment surgery; right eye.** The retinal detachment which originally stretched from the temporal superior fundus to the optic disc has now disappeared. The choroid is visible again. Broad arc-like scars lie under the plane of the retinal vessels and include the macula. Superior to this one can recognize a narrow attachment fold. Visual acuity: 5/15–5/10.

**Fig. 277. Condition after retinal detachment surgery; left eye.** 4 years ago there was a temporal inferior retinal detachment with a peripheral round hole, which was treated with trans-scleral ball-electrode diathermy. The retina is now attached. In the region of coagulation there are now irregular sharply demarcated scars through whose centres the pale sclera shimmers. At the superior edge of the scars is a fine radial folding of the retina.

**Fig. 278. Retrolental fibroplasia; left eye.** This 5-year-old patient has been under ophthalmological control since birth. He was a 7-months premature child and spent several weeks in an incubator. A few weeks after birth the right cornea clouded so that the fundus was not visible. On the left there is now an irregularly formed optic disc with an irregular vascular pattern. Nasally superior from the optic disc is a preretinal partially vascularized connective tissue band, running axially forwards into the vitreous. A larger venous branch accompanies this sail-like formation for a short distance, and then forms a hairpin bend back to the optic disc. Underneath the vitreous proliferation is a small choroiditic focus. Visual acuity: 5/10.

Tumours

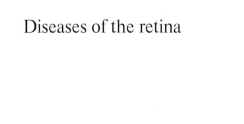

**Fig. 279. Retinoblastoma; left eye.** Amaurotic cat's eye in a 4-month-old infant. The yellowish coloured retina lies against the posterior surface of the lens. One can recognize several retinal vessels on the surface of the tumour.

**Fig. 280. Bourneville-Pringle's disease; right eye.** The disease was diagnosed 15 years ago in this 43-year-old patient who had typical changes of adenoma sebaceum on his face. Visual acuity was normal. A typical mulberry retinal tumour is situated temporally, superior to the optic disc.

**Fig. 281. Retinal angiomatosis; left eye.** This 20-year-old patient had always had poor vision on his left eye. One sees the typical picture of von Hippel-Lindau's disease: red tumour-like spherical aneurysmic vascular formations; as well as extreme varicosity of the temporal inferior vascular branches. Analogous angiomatous changes are frequently found in the cerebellum. In the present case there is also the onset of a stellate exudate figure in the macula, which resulted in progressive decrease in vision. In the region of the angiomatous knot one can see occasional haemorrhages. The tumour has been surrounded with light-coagulation foci as prophylaxis against the late complication of a tractional retinal detachment.

**Fig. 282 and 283. Leber's miliary aneurysms; right eye of the same patient.** In the region of the temporal superior vascular arc lie multiple microaneurysms of varying size mostly adjacent to the vessels, and situated in the centre of a wreath-like circinate retinopathy.

**Fig. 283 shows the findings 2½ months after treatment with Xenon-light-coagulation.** The foci are now sharply demarcated and of varying pigmentation, being partially confluent. One still finds a few delicate circinate-like changes, but the microaneurysms are no longer visible.

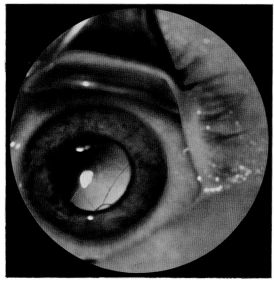

**279**

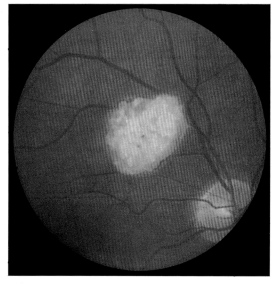

**280**

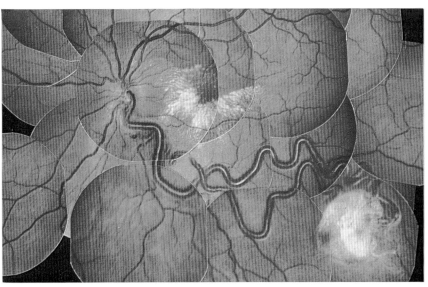

**281**

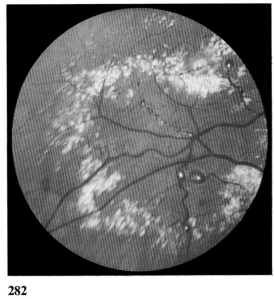

**282**

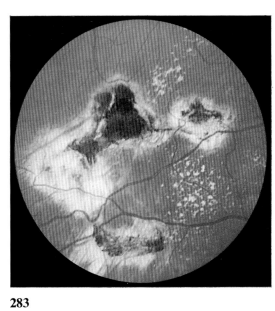

**283**

# Diseases of the choroid*

## Inflammatory lesions

* The vascular disorders of this part of the eye (choroidal sclerosis) have been dealt with under arteriosclerosis of the "retina".

135

**Fig. 284 and 285. Fresh (on the right), and old (on the left) central choroiditis.** Both eyes of the same 31-year-old patient. The right macula (Fig. 284) is the site of the relatively fresh, cloudy, diffuse, pale focus still indistinctly defined, in which however there is an onset of sharper demarcation as well as moderate pigmentation in several places. On the left side (Fig. 285) is an old choroiditis. There are pigmented, mainly finely spotted foci with rarification and in parts disappearance of the choroidal vessels between the optic disc and the macula and beyond. Visual acuity: right 5/25, left 5/20.

**Fig. 286. Fresh paracentral retinochoroiditis; right eye.** One sees a prominent yellowish white, indistinctly demarcated focus, with a chalk white centre temporal and superior to the optic disc in this 13-year-old patient. The course of the retinal vessels which appear either interrupted by this focus or flowing over it, justifies the description of a "pseudo-optic disc". Delicate radial folds of the retina are present inferior to this reaching the fovea. This zone is limited below by yellowish white foci.

**Fig. 287. No longer quite fresh, central choroiditis; left eye.** 7-year-old patient with a reflex-rich fundus. The central fundus is the site of an almost oval, large cockade-like focus. There are oedematous, blurred, paler areas alternating with delicate line and spot haemorrhages in its marginal zone. The almost triangular, irregularly pigmented change in the centre represents the onset of scarring. But even here there are still a few fine haemorrhages present.

**Fig. 288–290. Old central (paracentral) choroiditis.** The manifold appearance of these changes is seen in these 3 photographs. In Fig. 288 one recognizes a sharply demarcated dark focus surrounded by a definite boundary reflex, directly superior to the somewhat dark fovea centralis of this 25-year-old patient. In Fig. 289 are broader, on the whole less pigmented, irregular foci. Fig. 290 shows a massive, very intensely pigmented, central choroiditic scar lying in the middle of a sharply demarcated safron-yellow zone.

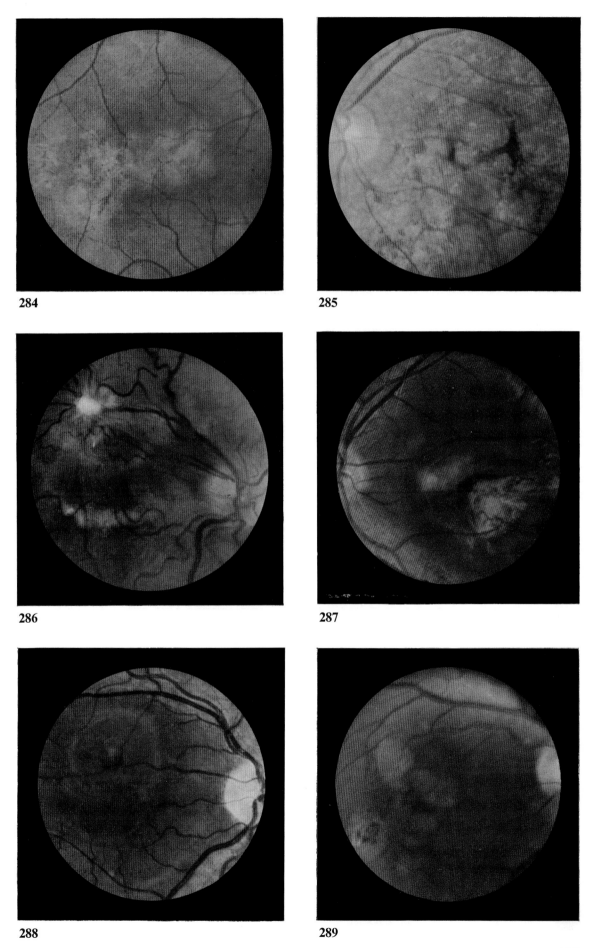

284

285

286

287

288

289

137

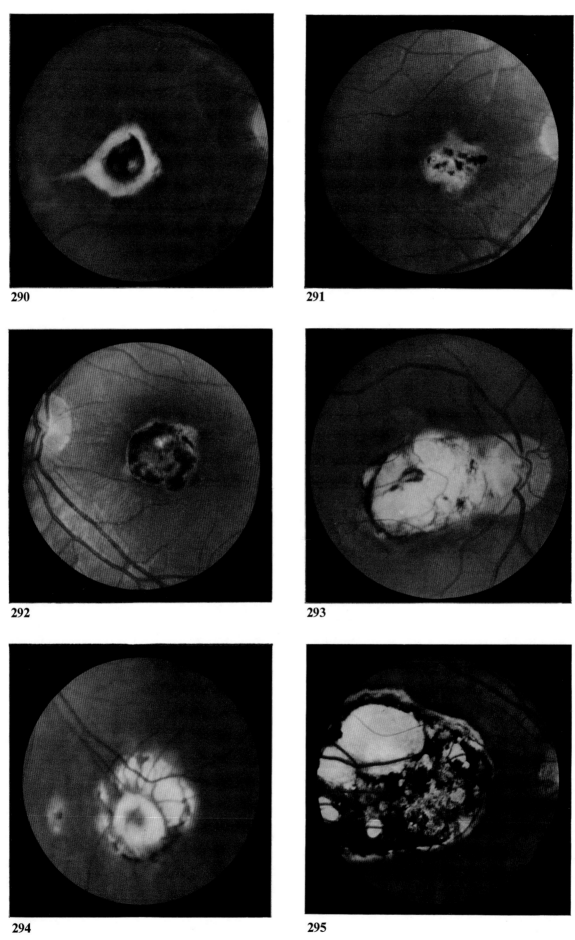

290

291

292

293

294

295

138

**Fig. 290  See page 136!**

**Fig. 291 and 292.  Congenital central choroiditis; right and left eye of the same 12-year-old patient.** On the right (Fig. 291), in the macula is an irregular old choroiditic scar the size of an optic disc, with irregular comparatively delicate pigmentation. On the left (Fig. 292), a considerably stronger pigmentation marks the aforegone central choroiditis. It is surrounded by a narrow depigmented halo. Recent experience of the last few years has shown that the picture of a congenital central choroiditis ("macula coloboma") can also be caused by an intrauterine toxoplasmosis infection. The intracerebral calcification, the neurological symptoms, as well as serological tests indicated such an aetiology in the present case.

**Fig. 293–295.  Further examples of congenital central choroditis in connatal toxoplasmosis.** Various large, healed and therefore sharply demarcated scars can be seen especially favouring the central fundus. The base of these scars is of varying pigmentation. Pigment can also be deposited in different forms and density at the margin of a focus, so that sometimes rosette-like pictures occur. Remarkable is the irregular course of the vessels still present within the scar tissue.

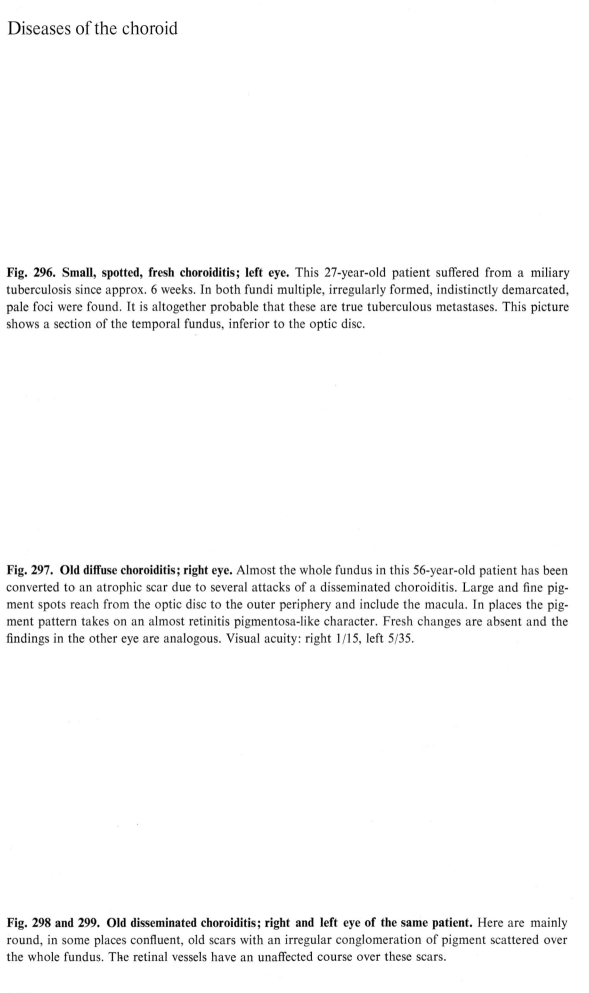

**Fig. 296. Small, spotted, fresh choroiditis; left eye.** This 27-year-old patient suffered from a miliary tuberculosis since approx. 6 weeks. In both fundi multiple, irregularly formed, indistinctly demarcated, pale foci were found. It is altogether probable that these are true tuberculous metastases. This picture shows a section of the temporal fundus, inferior to the optic disc.

**Fig. 297. Old diffuse choroiditis; right eye.** Almost the whole fundus in this 56-year-old patient has been converted to an atrophic scar due to several attacks of a disseminated choroiditis. Large and fine pigment spots reach from the optic disc to the outer periphery and include the macula. In places the pigment pattern takes on an almost retinitis pigmentosa-like character. Fresh changes are absent and the findings in the other eye are analogous. Visual acuity: right 1/15, left 5/35.

**Fig. 298 and 299. Old disseminated choroiditis; right and left eye of the same patient.** Here are mainly round, in some places confluent, old scars with an irregular conglomeration of pigment scattered over the whole fundus. The retinal vessels have an unaffected course over these scars.

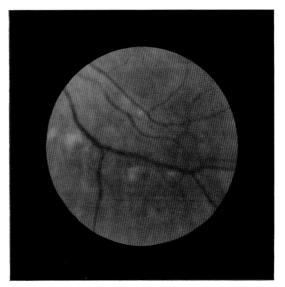

**296**

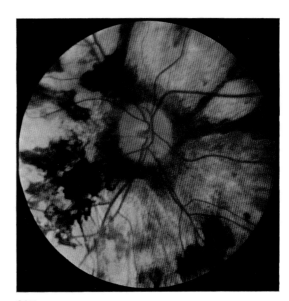

**297**

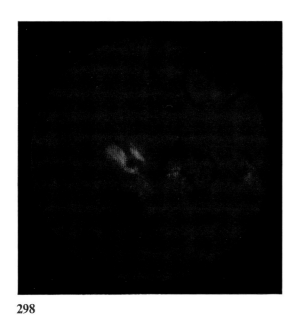

**298**

**299**

141

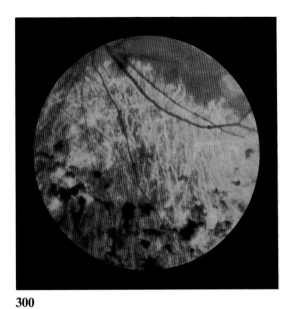

300

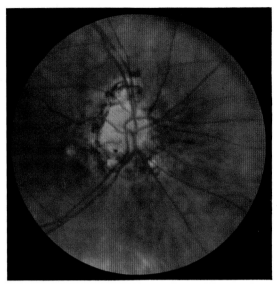

301

**Fig. 300. Old diffuse choroiditis; left eye.** Here in the centre are even larger islands of intact choroidal tissue. In the rest of the fundus however the choroid is almost completely destroyed, the choroidal vessels being replaced by pale bloodless strands. There are irregular conglomerations of pigment similar to a retinitis pigmentosa especially in the periphery.

**Fig. 301. Retino-choroiditis in congenital syphilis; right eye.** Here in the foreground of this 23-year-old patient's right fundus is a small old inflammation situated near the optic disc. Similar changes are in the outer periphery, the intermediate zone appearing normal in comparison. There is a distinct narrowing of the retinal vessels.

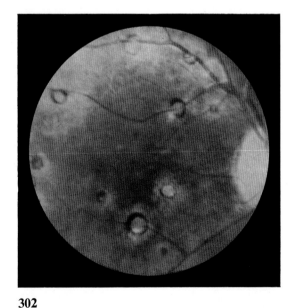

302

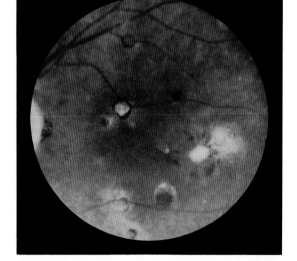

303

**Fig. 302 and 303. Retino-choroiditis in congenital syphilis; right and left eye of the same 8-year-old patient.** Here there are peculiar crater-like old foci scattered across the whole fundus. The centre of these lesions, which are mainly of similar size, is usually depigmented and is surrounded by a more or less complete, sharply demarcated pigmented circle. On the left side (Fig. 303), a small scar is also present in the centre of the fundus. Visual acuity: right 5/20, left 5/35.

142

Degenerative lesions*

* Compare also Fig. 247–250.

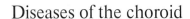

**Fig. 304. Peripapillary conus in myopia; right eye.** The circumpapillary myopic conus, a sharply demarcated absence of the choroid, is the result of retraction due to ectasia of the sclera. In this case there is still a single choroidal vessel visible at the superior optic disc margin. A further small accessory stretched area lies temporally and superiorly from the optic disc. The macula just visible in the left margin of the picture, shows pigmentation (so-called Fuchs' spot) as a remnant of an earlier haemorrhage. Visual acuity: 14,0 2/35 2/25.

**Fig. 305. Circular conus in pathologic (degenerative) myopia; right eye.** Widespread atrophy of the choroid which especially on the temporal side surrounds the optic disc, and almost reaches into the fovea; the macula being altered by pigmented and depigmented areas. There is slight blurring of the optic disc margins, with slight varicosity of the main retinal vessels (pseudoneuritis). Visual acuity: 20,0 5/20, 5/15.

**Fig. 306. Fundus in pathologic (degenerative) myopia; left eye.** The myopic stretched atrophic area includes the whole posterior section of the fundus. There is only a narrow irregular strip of intact choroid between the optic disc and the macula. Otherwise there are large stretches of choroidal atrophy with remarkably stretched retinal vessels. Visual acuity: 20,0 finger counting in 1 m.

**Fig. 307 and 308. Macular haemorrhage in myopia; right eye.** On the basis of the extreme stretching (refractive error – 16 dptr) there has been a sudden decrease in visual acuity in this 47-year-old patient 8 weeks ago. In the macula is a small haemorrhage (Fig. 307), which is situated cap-like on a pigmented zone, which has in all probability resulted from an earlier haemorrhage. Following a temporary improvement of visual acuity a renewed decrease occurred 28 days ago. The pigmented focus at the central fundus (Fig. 308) is now much larger. A fresh surface haemorrhage lies between the optic disc and the macula. Visual acuity: 16,0 1/20.

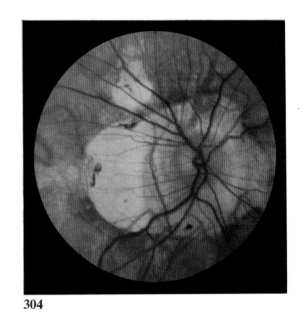

304

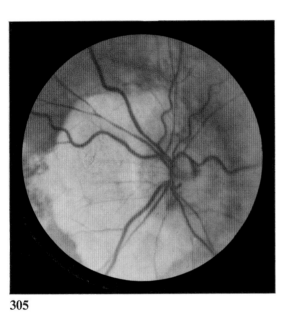

305

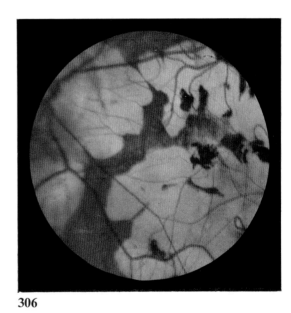

306

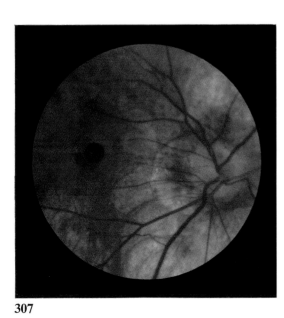

307

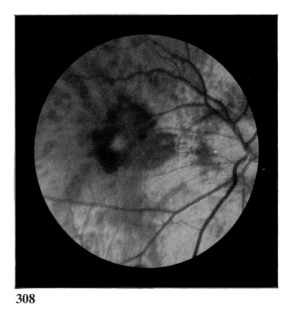

308

145

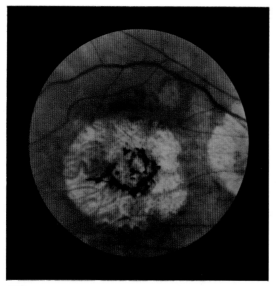

309

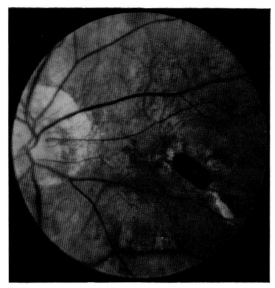

310

**Fig. 309 and 310. Pathologic (degenerative) myopia; right and left eye of the same 61-year-old patient.**
A bilateral myopic crescent is present as a sign of the myopia (visual acuity right: 17,0 5/35; left: 15,0
comb. – 0,75 cyl. A. 0° 5/25). On the right side (Fig. 309), there is also a widespread, depigmented focus
in the central fundus, in whose area obliterated choroidal vessels present as pale lines in between the
pigmented intervascular zones. In the middle of this area there is an almost circular pigmentation. On
the left (Fig. 310), is a Fuchs' spot in the form of a slanting oval pigmentation, with adjacent degenerative depigmented foci. Here also distinct tabulation of the mostly sclerotic, intervascular choroidal
spaces.

146

# Tumours

Diseases of the choroid

**Fig. 311. Melanoma of the choroid; left eye.** Here is a tumour that was opaque on trans-scleral illumination, which reaches the optic disc from inferiorly and includes the middle periphery. There is a fairly sharp demarcation to the adjacent attached retina. The course of the vessels show up the prominence clearly. At the inferior margin of the tumour as well as in its inferior third, one can recognize regressive changes in the form of yellowy white degenerative areas and delicate cloudy pale zones. An enucleation confirmed the diagnosis. Histologically tumour cells were already seen within the sclera.

**Fig. 312. Choroidal metastasis of a mammary carcinoma; right eye.** Carcinomas of the breast metastasize comparatively frequently to the choroid. This 35-year-old patient noticed a decrease in visual acuity 5 months after amputation of her breast. Inferior to the right optic disc is a low wavy retinal detachment with fine radial folds of the neighbouring retina.
This appeared to be the only metastasis as far as could be verified clinically. The patient refused an enucleation so long as there was no absolute proof that the fundus change was caused by a tumour. It was impossible to obtain material for cytological examination via needle puncture of the sclera. Therefore as an exception to the rule, an exploratory excision of choroidal tissue was undertaken at the site of the tumour. The histological sections showed a metastatic mammary carcinoma. 4 months later a similar solid retinal attachment due to a metastasis occurred in the other eye.

**Fig. 313. Circumscribed retinal detachment due to probable pulmonary cancer metastasis; left eye.** This 72-year-old patient had an inoperable bronchial carcinoma. Within a relatively short period of time a retinal detachment presented temporally, superior to the optic disc. Rapid spreading of the now quite bullous retinal detachment beyond the equator. The superior and temporal superior optic disc margins are obliterated, only the nasal inferior margin being still recognizable.

148

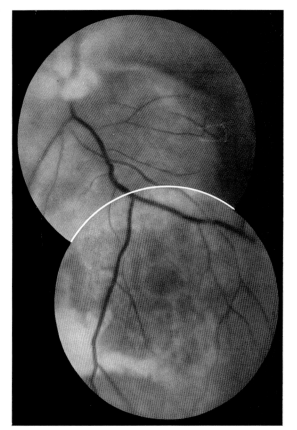

**311**

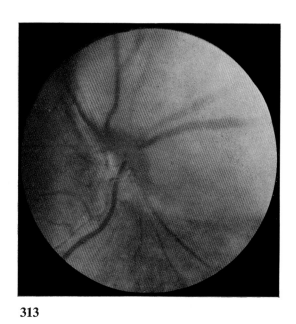

**312**

**313**

149

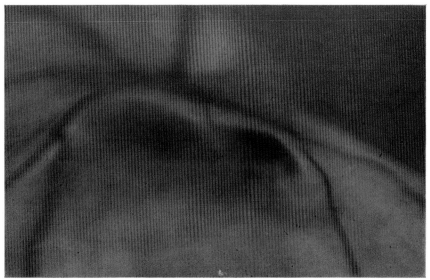

314

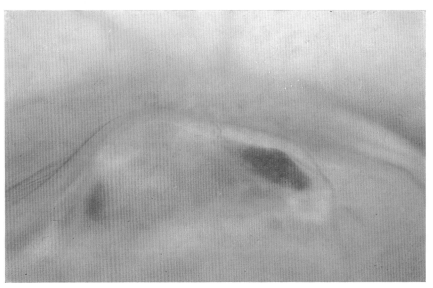

315

**Fig. 314 and 315. Malignant melanoma of the choroid; left eye.** Note the larger round prominent black tumour with a ridge encompassing the whole of the inferior circumference. The optic disc lies at a deeper plane and is indistinctly recognizable in the upper part of the picture. Photography with infra-red light (Fig. 315) shows the blackish-brown pigmentation of the tumour clearly differentiating it from a haemorrhage. Melanomas of this size are not infrequently responsible for a rise in intraocular tension. Ophthalmoscopically the dark colouring of a choroidal melanoma might not be seen due to the retroretinal transudate. However with the use of trans-scleral illumination such melanomas can be differentiated from ordinary retinal detachments.

150

Traumatic lesions

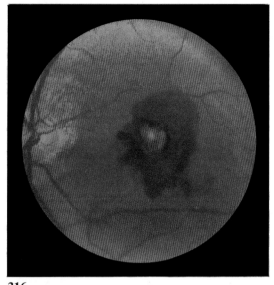

**316**

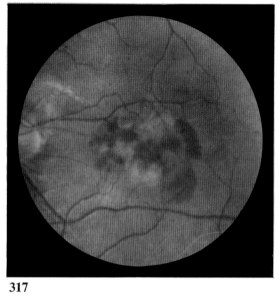

**317**

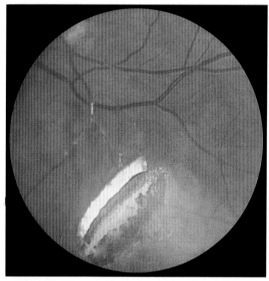

**318**

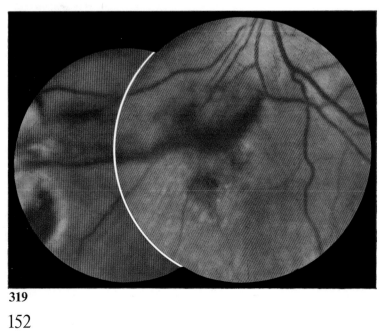

**319**

152

**Fig. 316 and 317. Haemorrhage at the central fundus after contusion of the eyeball; left eye.** 3 days after blunt trauma, surface haemorrhage in the macula region (Fig. 316). Superiorly and temporally the haemorrhage is crescent shaped, nasally and inferiorly it is irregularly demarcated. In the middle of the haemorrhage is an oval slate grey discolouration. Nasally and superior from this is a narrow pale line, reminiscent of a choroidal rupture. One week later (Fig. 317), the haemorrhage is partially resorbed. However there is now an increase in the dark focus in the central fundus. Visual acuity: 5/50.

**Fig. 318. Preretinal metallic foreign body; left eye.** This 8-year-old boy suffered a perforating injury while hammering a piece of metal during play. The silvery bright sharply-edged splinter lies in front of the retina and moves within the vitreous during eye movement. An arterial branch lying above it shows pale deposits and sheathing. Following extraction with a magnet, the wound healed without complications.

**Fig. 319. Condition after trans-scleral extraction of a foreign body; right eye.** 12 days ago a large iron splinter was situated directly preretinally in the temporal inferior area of the fundus. The sclera was incised in the centre of this area after blunt coagulation and the splinter extracted with a magnet. Now there is a flaglike haemorrhage preretinally inferior to the optic disc, with localised pigmentation directly inferior to it. Temporally and inferiorly one can recognise two still oedematous pale coagulation areas, the inferior one being covered to a greater extent by an arc-like haemorrhage.

**Fig. 320. Condition after trans-scleral extraction of a foreign body; right eye.** This patient suffered a penetrating iron-splinter injury 4 weeks ago. Immediate trans-scleral magnet extraction of the preretinal foreign body after a diathermy coagulation of the sclera in the neighbourhood was carried out. Here one sees a still relatively fresh, slightly blurred, coagulation area directly next to an already pigmented focus. At the nasal margin are a few haemorrhagic remnants.

**Fig. 321. Choroidal rupture; left eye.** 8 years ago this 10-year-old patient suffered a blunt trauma. Here is a broad arc-like rupture of the choroid starting at the optic disc and encompassing the macula with irregular pigmentation. At first this area was covered by a massive haemorrhage. Otherwise this is a youthful reflex-rich fundus.

**Fig. 322. Retinitis sclopedaria; left eye.** Gunshot wound of the left orbit ten years ago. The whole central fundus is intensely pale, and transformed into a connective tissue mass, with some strands occurring preretinally, and surrounded by spotty pigmentation.

**Fig. 323. Retinitis sclopedaria; left eye.** Condition after a gunshot wound through the temple during attempted suicide. Simple optic atrophy due to severance of the intraorbital optic nerve. Temporally and superior to the porcelain white optic disc is a widespread scarred area with pigmentation of varying density and distribution.

**Fig. 324. Retinitis sclopedaria after an old gunshot wound; left eye.** Here similar to the previous pictures is a widespread scarring inferior to the optic disc. The fundus is covered by a pale connective tissue mass including and beyond the equator. Temporally as well as superiorly to the optic disc, irregularly pigmented contusion areas over which occasional retinal vessels flow in an irregular manner.

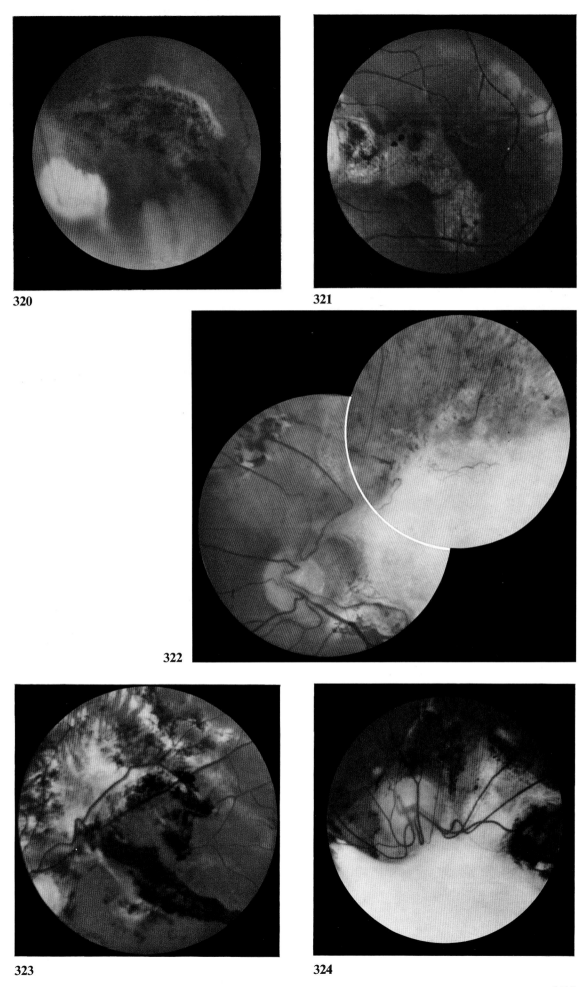

320

321

322

323

324

155

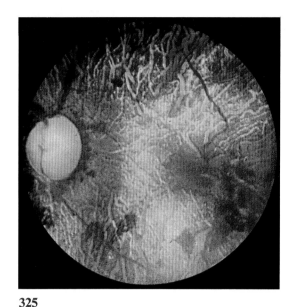

325

Fig. 325–327. Fundus in onchocercosis*.

**Fig. 325. So-called Ridley's fundus; left eye.**
This is the full picture of total retinal and choroidal sclerosis with optic atrophy. The exact mechanism of these changes which are naturally accompanied by extreme decrease in visual function is not exactly understood. It is probable that these changes are an expression of a local antigen-antibody reaction.

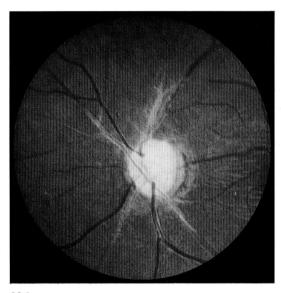

326

**Fig. 326. Fundus in onchocercosis; left eye.** Isolated optic atrophy with sharply defined margins and signs of a past periarteritis in the form of white sheathing of the larger arterial branches. On the venous side, one also recognizes similar, but far less marked changes.

**Fig. 327. Onchocercotic retinitis punctata albescens; right eye.** Here there are several pale foci of varying size which lie especially close together temporal to the macula. The fluorescenceangiography shows that these are defects of the pigment epithelium. Such fundus changes are most frequently seen in younger patients who have suffered an infection with onchocerca volvolus without other severe damage.

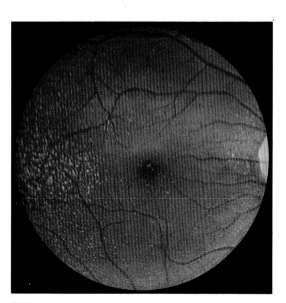

327

156

* We are indebted to Dr. Hans-Jürgen Trojan, eye specialist, Marburg/Lahn, formerly consultant of the eye clinic of the Centre Hospitalier Universitaire, Lome/Togo (West Africa) for kind permission to print these photographs.

Subject index

# Subject index

*The numbers given are figure numbers and not page numbers! The index is arranged so that findings specific to the choroid, the retina, the optic disc as well as the rabbit fundus can be found under these key-words.*

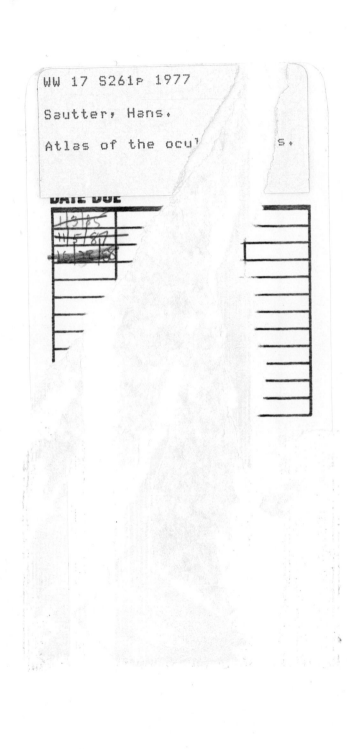